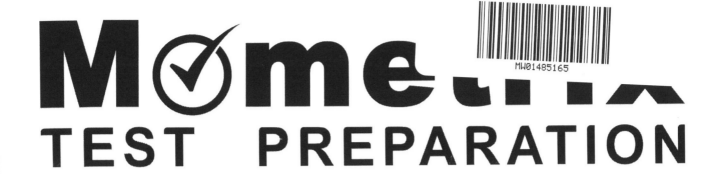

Clinical Nurse Leader
Exam Secrets
Study Guide

DEAR FUTURE EXAM SUCCESS STORY

First of all, **THANK YOU** for purchasing Mometrix study materials!

Second, congratulations! You are one of the few determined test-takers who are committed to doing whatever it takes to excel on your exam. **You have come to the right place.** We developed these study materials with one goal in mind: to deliver you the information you need in a format that's concise and easy to use.

In addition to optimizing your guide for the content of the test, we've outlined our recommended steps for breaking down the preparation process into small, attainable goals so you can make sure you stay on track.

We've also analyzed the entire test-taking process, identifying the most common pitfalls and showing how you can overcome them and be ready for any curveball the test throws you.

Standardized testing is one of the biggest obstacles on your road to success, which only increases the importance of doing well in the high-pressure, high-stakes environment of test day. Your results on this test could have a significant impact on your future, and this guide provides the information and practical advice to help you achieve your full potential on test day.

Your success is our success

We would love to hear from you! If you would like to share the story of your exam success or if you have any questions or comments in regard to our products, please contact us at **800-673-8175** or **support@mometrix.com**.

Thanks again for your business and we wish you continued success!

Sincerely,
The Mometrix Test Preparation Team

> **Need more help? Check out our flashcards at:**
> **http://mometrixflashcards.com/ClinicalNurseLeader**

TABLE OF CONTENTS

Introduction

Thank you for purchasing this resource! You have made the choice to prepare yourself for a test that could have a huge impact on your future, and this guide is designed to help you be fully ready for test day. Obviously, it's important to have a solid understanding of the test material, but you also need to be prepared for the unique environment and stressors of the test, so that you can perform to the best of your abilities.

For this purpose, the first section that appears in this guide is the **Secret Keys**. We've devoted countless hours to meticulously researching what works and what doesn't, and we've boiled down our findings to the five most impactful steps you can take to improve your performance on the test. We start at the beginning with study planning and move through the preparation process, all the way to the testing strategies that will help you get the most out of what you know when you're finally sitting in front of the test.

We recommend that you start preparing for your test as far in advance as possible. However, if you've bought this guide as a last-minute study resource and only have a few days before your test, we recommend that you skip over the first two Secret Keys since they address a long-term study plan.

If you struggle with **test anxiety**, we strongly encourage you to check out our recommendations for how you can overcome it. Test anxiety is a formidable foe, but it can be beaten, and we want to make sure you have the tools you need to defeat it.

Secret Key #1 – Plan Big, Study Small

There's a lot riding on your performance. If you want to ace this test, you're going to need to keep your skills sharp and the material fresh in your mind. You need a plan that lets you review everything you need to know while still fitting in your schedule. We'll break this strategy down into three categories.

Information Organization

Start with the information you already have: the official test outline. From this, you can make a complete list of all the concepts you need to cover before the test. Organize these concepts into groups that can be studied together, and create a list of any related vocabulary you need to learn so you can brush up on any difficult terms. You'll want to keep this vocabulary list handy once you actually start studying since you may need to add to it along the way.

Time Management

Once you have your set of study concepts, decide how to spread them out over the time you have left before the test. Break your study plan into small, clear goals so you have a manageable task for each day and know exactly what you're doing. Then just focus on one small step at a time. When you manage your time this way, you don't need to spend hours at a time studying. Studying a small block of content for a short period each day helps you retain information better and avoid stressing over how much you have left to do. You can relax knowing that you have a plan to cover everything in time. In order for this strategy to be effective though, you have to start studying early and stick to your schedule. Avoid the exhaustion and futility that comes from last-minute cramming!

Study Environment

The environment you study in has a big impact on your learning. Studying in a coffee shop, while probably more enjoyable, is not likely to be as fruitful as studying in a quiet room. It's important to keep distractions to a minimum. You're only planning to study for a short block of time, so make the most of it. Don't pause to check your phone or get up to find a snack. It's also important to **avoid multitasking**. Research has consistently shown that multitasking will make your studying dramatically less effective. Your study area should also be comfortable and well-lit so you don't have the distraction of straining your eyes or sitting on an uncomfortable chair.

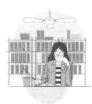 The time of day you study is also important. You want to be rested and alert. Don't wait until just before bedtime. Study when you'll be most likely to comprehend and remember. Even better, if you know what time of day your test will be, set that time aside for study. That way your brain will be used to working on that subject at that specific time and you'll have a better chance of recalling information.

Finally, it can be helpful to team up with others who are studying for the same test. Your actual studying should be done in as isolated an environment as possible, but the work of organizing the information and setting up the study plan can be divided up. In between study sessions, you can discuss with your teammates the concepts that you're all studying and quiz each other on the details. Just be sure that your teammates are as serious about the test as you are. If you find that your study time is being replaced with social time, you might need to find a new team.

Secret Key #2 – Make Your Studying Count

You're devoting a lot of time and effort to preparing for this test, so you want to be absolutely certain it will pay off. This means doing more than just reading the content and hoping you can remember it on test day. It's important to make every minute of study count. There are two main areas you can focus on to make your studying count.

Retention

It doesn't matter how much time you study if you can't remember the material. You need to make sure you are retaining the concepts. To check your retention of the information you're learning, try recalling it at later times with minimal prompting. Try carrying around flashcards and glance at one or two from time to time or ask a friend who's also studying for the test to quiz you.

To enhance your retention, look for ways to put the information into practice so that you can apply it rather than simply recalling it. If you're using the information in practical ways, it will be much easier to remember. Similarly, it helps to solidify a concept in your mind if you're not only reading it to yourself but also explaining it to someone else. Ask a friend to let you teach them about a concept you're a little shaky on (or speak aloud to an imaginary audience if necessary). As you try to summarize, define, give examples, and answer your friend's questions, you'll understand the concepts better and they will stay with you longer. Finally, step back for a big picture view and ask yourself how each piece of information fits with the whole subject. When you link the different concepts together and see them working together as a whole, it's easier to remember the individual components.

Finally, practice showing your work on any multi-step problems, even if you're just studying. Writing out each step you take to solve a problem will help solidify the process in your mind, and you'll be more likely to remember it during the test.

Modality

Modality simply refers to the means or method by which you study. Choosing a study modality that fits your own individual learning style is crucial. No two people learn best in exactly the same way, so it's important to know your strengths and use them to your advantage.

For example, if you learn best by visualization, focus on visualizing a concept in your mind and draw an image or a diagram. Try color-coding your notes, illustrating them, or creating symbols that will trigger your mind to recall a learned concept. If you learn best by hearing or discussing information, find a study partner who learns the same way or read aloud to yourself. Think about how to put the information in your own words. Imagine that you are giving a lecture on the topic and record yourself so you can listen to it later.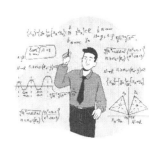

For any learning style, flashcards can be helpful. Organize the information so you can take advantage of spare moments to review. Underline key words or phrases. Use different colors for different categories. Mnemonic devices (such as creating a short list in which every item starts with the same letter) can also help with retention. Find what works best for you and use it to store the information in your mind most effectively and easily.

3

Secret Key #3 – Practice the Right Way

Your success on test day depends not only on how many hours you put into preparing, but also on whether you prepared the right way. It's good to check along the way to see if your studying is paying off. One of the most effective ways to do this is by taking practice tests to evaluate your progress. Practice tests are useful because they show exactly where you need to improve. Every time you take a practice test, pay special attention to these three groups of questions:

- The questions you got wrong
- The questions you had to guess on, even if you guessed right
- The questions you found difficult or slow to work through

This will show you exactly what your weak areas are, and where you need to devote more study time. Ask yourself why each of these questions gave you trouble. Was it because you didn't understand the material? Was it because you didn't remember the vocabulary? Do you need more repetitions on this type of question to build speed and confidence? Dig into those questions and figure out how you can strengthen your weak areas as you go back to review the material.

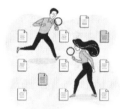 Additionally, many practice tests have a section explaining the answer choices. It can be tempting to read the explanation and think that you now have a good understanding of the concept. However, an explanation likely only covers part of the question's broader context. Even if the explanation makes perfect sense, **go back and investigate** every concept related to the question until you're positive you have a thorough understanding.

As you go along, keep in mind that the practice test is just that: practice. Memorizing these questions and answers will not be very helpful on the actual test because it is unlikely to have any of the same exact questions. If you only know the right answers to the sample questions, you won't be prepared for the real thing. **Study the concepts** until you understand them fully, and then you'll be able to answer any question that shows up on the test.

It's important to wait on the practice tests until you're ready. If you take a test on your first day of study, you may be overwhelmed by the amount of material covered and how much you need to learn. Work up to it gradually.

On test day, you'll need to be prepared for answering questions, managing your time, and using the test-taking strategies you've learned. It's a lot to balance, like a mental marathon that will have a big impact on your future. Like training for a marathon, you'll need to start slowly and work your way up. When test day arrives, you'll be ready.

Start with the strategies you've read in the first two Secret Keys—plan your course and study in the way that works best for you. If you have time, consider using multiple study resources to get different approaches to the same concepts. It can be helpful to see difficult concepts from more than one angle. Then find a good source for practice tests. Many times, the test website will suggest potential study resources or provide sample tests.

4

Practice Test Strategy

If you're able to find at least three practice tests, we recommend this strategy:

UNTIMED AND OPEN-BOOK PRACTICE

Take the first test with no time constraints and with your notes and study guide handy. Take your time and focus on applying the strategies you've learned.

TIMED AND OPEN-BOOK PRACTICE

Take the second practice test open-book as well, but set a timer and practice pacing yourself to finish in time.

TIMED AND CLOSED-BOOK PRACTICE

Take any other practice tests as if it were test day. Set a timer and put away your study materials. Sit at a table or desk in a quiet room, imagine yourself at the testing center, and answer questions as quickly and accurately as possible.

Keep repeating timed and closed-book tests on a regular basis until you run out of practice tests or it's time for the actual test. Your mind will be ready for the schedule and stress of test day, and you'll be able to focus on recalling the material you've learned.

Secret Key #4 – Pace Yourself

Once you're fully prepared for the material on the test, your biggest challenge on test day will be managing your time. Just knowing that the clock is ticking can make you panic even if you have plenty of time left. Work on pacing yourself so you can build confidence against the time constraints of the exam. Pacing is a difficult skill to master, especially in a high-pressure environment, so **practice is vital**.

Set time expectations for your pace based on how much time is available. For example, if a section has 60 questions and the time limit is 30 minutes, you know you have to average 30 seconds or less per question in order to answer them all. Although 30 seconds is the hard limit, set 25 seconds per question as your goal, so you reserve extra time to spend on harder questions. When you budget extra time for the harder questions, you no longer have any reason to stress when those questions take longer to answer.

Don't let this time expectation distract you from working through the test at a calm, steady pace, but keep it in mind so you don't spend too much time on any one question. Recognize that taking extra time on one question you don't understand may keep you from answering two that you do understand later in the test. If your time limit for a question is up and you're still not sure of the answer, mark it and move on, and come back to it later if the time and the test format allow. If the testing format doesn't allow you to return to earlier questions, just make an educated guess; then put it out of your mind and move on.

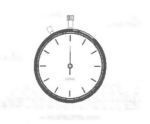

On the easier questions, be careful not to rush. It may seem wise to hurry through them so you have more time for the challenging ones, but it's not worth missing one if you know the concept and just didn't take the time to read the question fully. Work efficiently but make sure you understand the question and have looked at all of the answer choices, since more than one may seem right at first.

Even if you're paying attention to the time, you may find yourself a little behind at some point. You should speed up to get back on track, but do so wisely. Don't panic; just take a few seconds less on each question until you're caught up. Don't guess without thinking, but do look through the answer choices and eliminate any you know are wrong. If you can get down to two choices, it is often worthwhile to guess from those. Once you've chosen an answer, move on and don't dwell on any that you skipped or had to hurry through. If a question was taking too long, chances are it was one of the harder ones, so you weren't as likely to get it right anyway.

On the other hand, if you find yourself getting ahead of schedule, it may be beneficial to slow down a little. The more quickly you work, the more likely you are to make a careless mistake that will affect your score. You've budgeted time for each question, so don't be afraid to spend that time. Practice an efficient but careful pace to get the most out of the time you have.

6

Secret Key #5 – Have a Plan for Guessing

When you're taking the test, you may find yourself stuck on a question. Some of the answer choices seem better than others, but you don't see the one answer choice that is obviously correct. What do you do?

The scenario described above is very common, yet most test takers have not effectively prepared for it. Developing and practicing a plan for guessing may be one of the single most effective uses of your time as you get ready for the exam.

In developing your plan for guessing, there are three questions to address:

- When should you start the guessing process?
- How should you narrow down the choices?
- Which answer should you choose?

When to Start the Guessing Process

Unless your plan for guessing is to select C every time (which, despite its merits, is not what we recommend), you need to leave yourself enough time to apply your answer elimination strategies. Since you have a limited amount of time for each question, that means that if you're going to give yourself the best shot at guessing correctly, you have to decide quickly whether or not you will guess.

Of course, the best-case scenario is that you don't have to guess at all, so first, see if you can answer the question based on your knowledge of the subject and basic reasoning skills. Focus on the key words in the question and try to jog your memory of related topics. Give yourself a chance to bring the knowledge to mind, but once you realize that you don't have (or you can't access) the knowledge you need to answer the question, it's time to start the guessing process.

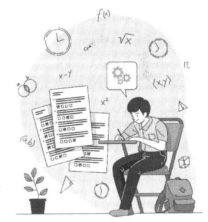

It's almost always better to start the guessing process too early than too late. It only takes a few seconds to remember something and answer the question from knowledge. Carefully eliminating wrong answer choices takes longer. Plus, going through the process of eliminating answer choices can actually help jog your memory.

Summary: Start the guessing process as soon as you decide that you can't answer the question based on your knowledge.

7

How to Narrow Down the Choices

The next chapter in this book (**Test-Taking Strategies**) includes a wide range of strategies for how to approach questions and how to look for answer choices to eliminate. You will definitely want to read those carefully, practice them, and figure out which ones work best for you. Here though, we're going to address a mindset rather than a particular strategy.

Your odds of guessing an answer correctly depend on how many options you are choosing from.

Number of options left	5	4	3	2	1
Odds of guessing correctly	20%	25%	33%	50%	100%

You can see from this chart just how valuable it is to be able to eliminate incorrect answers and make an educated guess, but there are two things that many test takers do that cause them to miss out on the benefits of guessing:

- Accidentally eliminating the correct answer
- Selecting an answer based on an impression

We'll look at the first one here, and the second one in the next section.

To avoid accidentally eliminating the correct answer, we recommend a thought exercise called **the $5 challenge**. In this challenge, you only eliminate an answer choice from contention if you are willing to bet $5 on it being wrong. Why $5? Five dollars is a small but not insignificant amount of money. It's an amount you could afford to lose but wouldn't want to throw away. And while losing

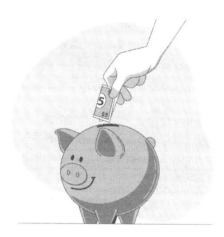

$5 once might not hurt too much, doing it twenty times will set you back $100. In the same way, each small decision you make—eliminating a choice here, guessing on a question there—won't by itself impact your score very much, but when you put them all together, they can make a big difference. By holding each answer choice elimination decision to a higher standard, you can reduce the risk of accidentally eliminating the correct answer.

The $5 challenge can also be applied in a positive sense: If you are willing to bet $5 that an answer choice *is* correct, go ahead and mark it as correct.

Summary: Only eliminate an answer choice if you are willing to bet $5 that it is wrong.

8

Which Answer to Choose

You're taking the test. You've run into a hard question and decided you'll have to guess. You've eliminated all the answer choices you're willing to bet $5 on. Now you have to pick an answer. Why do we even need to talk about this? Why can't you just pick whichever one you feel like when the time comes?

The answer to these questions is that if you don't come into the test with a plan, you'll rely on your impression to select an answer choice, and if you do that, you risk falling into a trap. The test writers know that everyone who takes their test will be guessing on some of the questions, so they intentionally write wrong answer choices to seem plausible. You still have to pick an answer though, and if the wrong answer choices are designed to look right, how can you ever be sure that you're not falling for their trap? The best solution we've found to this dilemma is to take the decision out of your hands entirely. Here is the process we recommend:

Once you've eliminated any choices that you are confident (willing to bet $5) are wrong, select the first remaining choice as your answer.

Whether you choose to select the first remaining choice, the second, or the last, the important thing is that you use some preselected standard. Using this approach guarantees that you will not be enticed into selecting an answer choice that looks right, because you are not basing your decision on how the answer choices look.

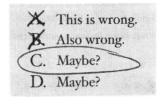

This is not meant to make you question your knowledge. Instead, it is to help you recognize the difference between your knowledge and your impressions. There's a huge difference between thinking an answer is right because of what you know, and thinking an answer is right because it looks or sounds like it should be right.

Summary: To ensure that your selection is appropriately random, make a predetermined selection from among all answer choices you have not eliminated.

Test-Taking Strategies

This section contains a list of test-taking strategies that you may find helpful as you work through the test. By taking what you know and applying logical thought, you can maximize your chances of answering any question correctly!

It is very important to realize that every question is different and every person is different: no single strategy will work on every question, and no single strategy will work for every person. That's why we've included all of them here, so you can try them out and determine which ones work best for different types of questions and which ones work best for you.

Question Strategies

⊘ READ CAREFULLY

Read the question and the answer choices carefully. Don't miss the question because you misread the terms. You have plenty of time to read each question thoroughly and make sure you understand what is being asked. Yet a happy medium must be attained, so don't waste too much time. You must read carefully and efficiently.

⊘ CONTEXTUAL CLUES

Look for contextual clues. If the question includes a word you are not familiar with, look at the immediate context for some indication of what the word might mean. Contextual clues can often give you all the information you need to decipher the meaning of an unfamiliar word. Even if you can't determine the meaning, you may be able to narrow down the possibilities enough to make a solid guess at the answer to the question.

⊘ PREFIXES

If you're having trouble with a word in the question or answer choices, try dissecting it. Take advantage of every clue that the word might include. Prefixes can be a huge help. Usually, they allow you to determine a basic meaning. *Pre-* means before, *post-* means after, *pro-* is positive, *de-* is negative. From prefixes, you can get an idea of the general meaning of the word and try to put it into context.

⊘ HEDGE WORDS

Watch out for critical hedge words, such as *likely, may, can, sometimes, often, almost, mostly, usually, generally, rarely,* and *sometimes.* Question writers insert these hedge phrases to cover every possibility. Often an answer choice will be wrong simply because it leaves no room for exception. Be on guard for answer choices that have definitive words such as *exactly* and *always.*

⊘ SWITCHBACK WORDS

Stay alert for *switchbacks.* These are the words and phrases frequently used to alert you to shifts in thought. The most common switchback words are *but, although,* and *however.* Others include *nevertheless, on the other hand, even though, while, in spite of, despite,* and *regardless of.* Switchback words are important to catch because they can change the direction of the question or an answer choice.

10

⊘ Face Value

When in doubt, use common sense. Accept the situation in the problem at face value. Don't read too much into it. These problems will not require you to make wild assumptions. If you have to go beyond creativity and warp time or space in order to have an answer choice fit the question, then you should move on and consider the other answer choices. These are normal problems rooted in reality. The applicable relationship or explanation may not be readily apparent, but it is there for you to figure out. Use your common sense to interpret anything that isn't clear.

Answer Choice Strategies

⊘ Answer Selection

The most thorough way to pick an answer choice is to identify and eliminate wrong answers until only one is left, then confirm it is the correct answer. Sometimes an answer choice may immediately seem right, but be careful. The test writers will usually put more than one reasonable answer choice on each question, so take a second to read all of them and make sure that the other choices are not equally obvious. As long as you have time left, it is better to read every answer choice than to pick the first one that looks right without checking the others.

⊘ Answer Choice Families

An answer choice family consists of two (in rare cases, three) answer choices that are very similar in construction and cannot all be true at the same time. If you see two answer choices that are direct opposites or parallels, one of them is usually the correct answer. For instance, if one answer choice says that quantity x increases and another either says that quantity x decreases (opposite) or says that quantity y increases (parallel), then those answer choices would fall into the same family. An answer choice that doesn't match the construction of the answer choice family is more likely to be incorrect. Most questions will not have answer choice families, but when they do appear, you should be prepared to recognize them.

⊘ Eliminate Answers

Eliminate answer choices as soon as you realize they are wrong, but make sure you consider all possibilities. If you are eliminating answer choices and realize that the last one you are left with is also wrong, don't panic. Start over and consider each choice again. There may be something you missed the first time that you will realize on the second pass.

⊘ Avoid Fact Traps

Don't be distracted by an answer choice that is factually true but doesn't answer the question. You are looking for the choice that answers the question. Stay focused on what the question is asking for so you don't accidentally pick an answer that is true but incorrect. Always go back to the question and make sure the answer choice you've selected actually answers the question and is not merely a true statement.

⊘ Extreme Statements

In general, you should avoid answers that put forth extreme actions as standard practice or proclaim controversial ideas as established fact. An answer choice that states the "process should be used in certain situations, if..." is much more likely to be correct than one that states the "process should be discontinued completely." The first is a calm rational statement and doesn't even make a definitive, uncompromising stance, using a hedge word *if* to provide wiggle room, whereas the second choice is far more extreme.

11

⊘ Benchmark

As you read through the answer choices and you come across one that seems to answer the question well, mentally select that answer choice. This is not your final answer, but it's the one that will help you evaluate the other answer choices. The one that you selected is your benchmark or standard for judging each of the other answer choices. Every other answer choice must be compared to your benchmark. That choice is correct until proven otherwise by another answer choice beating it. If you find a better answer, then that one becomes your new benchmark. Once you've decided that no other choice answers the question as well as your benchmark, you have your final answer.

⊘ Predict the Answer

Before you even start looking at the answer choices, it is often best to try to predict the answer. When you come up with the answer on your own, it is easier to avoid distractions and traps because you will know exactly what to look for. The right answer choice is unlikely to be word-for-word what you came up with, but it should be a close match. Even if you are confident that you have the right answer, you should still take the time to read each option before moving on.

General Strategies

⊘ Tough Questions

If you are stumped on a problem or it appears too hard or too difficult, don't waste time. Move on! Remember though, if you can quickly check for obviously incorrect answer choices, your chances of guessing correctly are greatly improved. Before you completely give up, at least try to knock out a couple of possible answers. Eliminate what you can and then guess at the remaining answer choices before moving on.

⊘ Check Your Work

Since you will probably not know every term listed and the answer to every question, it is important that you get credit for the ones that you do know. Don't miss any questions through careless mistakes. If at all possible, try to take a second to look back over your answer selection and make sure you've selected the correct answer choice and haven't made a costly careless mistake (such as marking an answer choice that you didn't mean to mark). This quick double check should more than pay for itself in caught mistakes for the time it costs.

⊘ Pace Yourself

It's easy to be overwhelmed when you're looking at a page full of questions; your mind is confused and full of random thoughts, and the clock is ticking down faster than you would like. Calm down and maintain the pace that you have set for yourself. Especially as you get down to the last few minutes of the test, don't let the small numbers on the clock make you panic. As long as you are on track by monitoring your pace, you are guaranteed to have time for each question.

⊘ Don't Rush

It is very easy to make errors when you are in a hurry. Maintaining a fast pace in answering questions is pointless if it makes you miss questions that you would have gotten right otherwise. Test writers like to include distracting information and wrong answers that seem right. Taking a little extra time to avoid careless mistakes can make all the difference in your test score. Find a pace that allows you to be confident in the answers that you select.

⊘ KEEP MOVING

Panicking will not help you pass the test, so do your best to stay calm and keep moving. Taking deep breaths and going through the answer elimination steps you practiced can help to break through a stress barrier and keep your pace.

Final Notes

The combination of a solid foundation of content knowledge and the confidence that comes from practicing your plan for applying that knowledge is the key to maximizing your performance on test day. As your foundation of content knowledge is built up and strengthened, you'll find that the strategies included in this chapter become more and more effective in helping you quickly sift through the distractions and traps of the test to isolate the correct answer.

Now that you're preparing to move forward into the test content chapters of this book, be sure to keep your goal in mind. As you read, think about how you will be able to apply this information on the test. If you've already seen sample questions for the test and you have an idea of the question format and style, try to come up with questions of your own that you can answer based on what you're reading. This will give you valuable practice applying your knowledge in the same ways you can expect to on test day.

Good luck and good studying!

Nursing Leadership

Horizontal Leadership

EFFECTIVE NURSING GROUP LEADERS

Effective nursing group leaders possess several qualities in common to be able to manage a group and help it successfully achieve its goals. Effective group leaders must have the ability to organize information, particularly when data are presented in a disorganized manner. They must be able to listen actively to team members and be able to understand nonverbal cues. Nurse leaders must give appropriate and timely feedback to participants who spend time performing or presenting their parts of the work of the team. This helps the group to sort through information that works toward the team's objectives as well as those data that still need to be obtained or reinforced. Overall, effective group leaders must be aware of what is going on within the group and have a passion for the group's goals, being willing to take the time to listen, review data, organize information, and manage the group's efforts.

HORIZONTAL AND VERTICAL LEADERSHIP

With **vertical leadership**, a hierarchical system is in place with management at the top and those below in descending order with a clearly outlined chain of command. Generally, authority and decision-making rests with those at the top of the chain of command, and while the leader may seek input from others, they do not have a say in the final decision. The CNL's role depends on where in the hierarchy the CNL falls. Most control is with clinical care rather than management issues.

With **horizontal leadership**, the chain of command is limited, and department managers are fairly autonomous in making decisions. Decisions are reached through collaboration, and all members are encouraged to contribute ideas and innovations. As a leader, the CNL would work closely with staff members on clinical issues and may manage scheduling, allocation of resources, and budgeting for the unit, but with input from staff members.

LEADERSHIP STYLES

Leadership styles often influence the perception of leadership values and commitment to collaboration. There are a number of different leadership styles:

- **Charismatic** – Depends upon personal charisma to influence people, and may be very persuasive, but this type leader may engage "followers" and relate to one group rather than the organization at large, limiting effectiveness.
- **Bureaucratic** – Follows organization rules exactly and expects everyone else to do so. This is most effective in handling cash flow or managing work in dangerous work environments. This type of leadership may engender respect but may not be conducive to change.
- **Autocratic** – Makes decisions independently and strictly enforces rules, but team members often feel left out of process and may not be supportive. This type of leadership is most effective in crisis situations, but may have difficulty gaining commitment of staff.
- **Consultative** – Presents a decision and welcomes input and questions although decisions rarely change. This type of leadership is most effective when gaining the support of staff is critical to the success of proposed changes.

15

- **Participatory** – Presents a potential decision and then makes final decision based on input from staff or teams. This type of leadership is time-consuming and may result in compromises that are not wholly satisfactory to management or staff, but this process is motivating to staff who feel their expertise is valued.
- **Democratic** – Presents a problem and asks staff or teams to arrive at a solution although the leader usually makes the final decision. This type of leadership may delay decision-making, but staff and teams are often more committed to the solutions because of their input.
- **Laissez-faire (free rein)** – Exerts little direct control but allows employees/ teams to make decisions with little interference. This may be effective leadership if teams are highly skilled and motivated; but, in many cases, this type of leadership is the product of poor management skills and little is accomplished because of this lack of leadership.

Leadership Theories

Theories are systems of ideas about topics that are based on related evidence or principles. Within health care, theories are developed in relation to situations, including those that explain behavior, symptom development, or influences on the health of patients. Nurses use theories to better understand the behavior of patients and to know how to interact with patients in response to this behavior. Theories are an important part of education because they help practitioners set goals for what patients should understand or to facilitate outcomes better. Many educational delivery programs are based on theories because they can explain behaviors and responses of patients, which help practitioners to identify those educational methods that may be successful and to which methods patients may be resistant.

HILDEGARD E. PEPLAU'S THEORY OF INTERPERSONAL RELATIONS

Hildegard E. Peplau's **Theory of Interpersonal Relations** focuses on the relationship between the patient and the nurse. The basic theory consists of four phases, which can be applied to clinical nursing practice.

1. Phase one is the **orientation phase**, in which the patient seeks help through appointments, treatment sessions, or other interventions from the nurse. During this phase, the nurse determines the patient's need for assistance.
2. The second phase is **identification**, in which the nurse helps the patient to identify who can help, and together the nurse and the patient set goals for care.
3. In the **exploitation phase**, the patient receives the care from the nurse.
4. In the **resolution phase**, all care is completed, and the patient–nurse relationship ends.

TRANSFORMATIONAL LEADERSHIP THEORY

Transformational leadership theory (Burns, Bass) stresses the impact that leaders can have to facilitate change. Instead of a transactional style of leadership in which change is brought about through a system of rewards and punishments (or withholding of rewards), a transformational leader leads change through showing respect and consideration for individuals, challenging them intellectually, and inspiring and influencing them. Transformational leaders are often personally charismatic and tend to lead through example rather than control. As a transformational leader, the CNL identifies those things that need change and old methods that are inefficient and works with other members of the team to motivate them and help them to find solutions and new and more efficient methods of doing things. The transformational leader provides a sense of direction and empowers others while focusing on collective purpose and pride in work and achievement, motivating others to do their best.

CHANGE THEORY CONCEPTS

Change theory was developed by Kurt Lewin to describe the process of eliminating unhealthy habits or behaviors and replacing them with new healthy ones.

- Change theory consists of **three phases**: unfreezing, which involves letting go of old habits; change, which involves making the change to a healthier habit; and refreezing, which permanently implements the change as a new habit.
- **Driving forces** are those that support change or push patients toward understanding necessary changes. For example, if patients want to quit smoking, driving forces may be their desire for better health and to breathe easier.
- **Restraining forces** are those that work against driving forces to inhibit change. In the example of patients who want to quit smoking, a restraining force may be that patients live with people who smoke, where it would be too difficult to quit under those circumstances.
- **Equilibrium** occurs when driving and restraining forces are of equal strength.

MASLOW'S HIERARCY OF NEEDS

Nurses must ensure that patients' needs are being met to determine appropriate outcomes. **Maslow's hierarchy of needs** helps nurses to determine priorities for patients based on whether their needs are fulfilled. The base of the hierarchy is physiological needs, the second level is safety, the third is psychological or emotional needs, the fourth level is self-esteem, and the top tier is self-actualization. Nurses should make goals that coincide with where patients are on the hierarchy and then work to reach those goals while fulfilling other needs on the hierarchy. For example, nurses should first meet the physiological needs for food, water, sleep, and treatment before focusing on outcomes in the higher levels on the hierarchy.

SYSTEMS THINKING

Systems thinking is concerned with how each part of the environment comes together to affect the other parts and the overall system. Nurses who practice systems thinking consider those processes that affect each other in nursing care. Processes, such as risk assessments, medical errors, staffing issues, and treatment compliance can all be analyzed as part of systems thinking. When nurses practice systems thinking, the outcomes can benefit patients, nurses, and the organization as a whole. For example, if nurses practice systems thinking about use of narcotics within the health care environment, they may consider the policies related to administration, analyze patient, outcomes when taking these medications, and assess for risks associated with use. If any area needs to be changed as a result of the nurses' analyses, the team works together to implement new structure. This ultimately benefits the patients receiving the medication as well as the nurses administering it, maintaining safety and quality within the environment.

SYSTEMS THINKING VS. THINKING ABOUT INDIVIDUAL CIRCUMSTANCES

Systems thinking differ from traditional thinking about individual circumstances as it considers the larger picture of the organization. Systems thinking involve consideration of the interconnected groups and frameworks that go together to make the unit or organization run smoothly. Nurses who use systems thinking consider several angles when tackling issues as well as how each of these approaches affects each other. Systems thinking can be said to be a circular process, in which systems interact and support each other. Alternatively, an individualist approach considers how to solve one issue at a time based on the specific information at hand. Individualistic thinking is more of a linear process, which considers how one aspect of a situation affects the next.

APPLYING SYSTEMS THINKING APPROACH TO STAFFING ISSUES

The **staffing issues** in nursing are commonplace in many health care organizations that try to maintain schedules. When implementing systems thinking toward the challenge of staffing issues, the organization must determine what practices are important to continue and what practices should be stopped. The organization also needs to consider how its actions will affect nurses in all units of the hospital or even those in the community who are aware of its efforts to hire and retain nurses. Systems thinking also involve consideration of the future effects of how staffing issues are managed. Certain actions must be considered as more than temporary measures to fill holes or maintain patient–staff ratios at the last minute.

IMPORTANCE OF COLLABORATION FOR SYSTEMS THINKING

Systems thinking requires **collaboration** with an interdisciplinary team who can provide varying viewpoints to work together to solve current problems. Because systems thinking requires looking at a situation and how it affects other parts of the organization as well as how other systems affect the situation, a team approach with varying points of view is necessary to determine who is affected and how to handle it. Multiple viewpoints from an interdisciplinary team also provide resources from different areas, which can be used to solve problems. The team works together to see how their perspectives interact in a specific situation, bringing ideas and expertise together to form potential solutions.

COMPLEXITY THEORY

The **complexity theory** was developed from systems theory and proposes that a complex system/organization comprises many different elements and levels, like a complex living organism rather than a machine, and that there is an intrinsic order to a complex system, even though it may not be obvious. According to this theory, the behavior of the group/system and the ability to self-organize as a whole may be different from individual behavior and results from interactions and adaptation. Therefore, it is difficult to determine how any change in a system will affect outcomes because outcomes are so dependent on the interactions that occur and cannot be predicted. The theory includes the idea that systems tend to organize themselves if left to function without extensive control and continually adapt to change. This theory recognizes that a system may have a built-in order (hierarchical decision making) but that no one can really maintain complete control as the system will evolve in its own way.

RATIONAL ORGANIZATIONAL THEORY

Rational Organizational Theory (Taylor) provides a framework and structure for making decisions and focuses on the logical/rational decisions necessary to reach organizational goals. Clearly outlined steps are used in the decision-making process in order to improve efficiency: determine goals and desired outcomes, collect data, brainstorm to determine possible actions, determine positive and negatives for each action, reach a decision, implement changes, and analyze outcomes. While having a clearly outlined process may simplify decision-making, an over-reliance on process may result in overlooking ethical and human issues. Rational organizational theory is based on scientific management and is generally applied to a hierarchical system in which the organization has specific goals and each individual has clearly-defined roles and responsibilities in achieving those goals. There may be little room for individual innovation or creativity as workers may have no control over processes, which are developed to maximize productivity.

CONTINGENCY THEORY

Contingency Theory is a theory of organizational behavior that states that there is no one best method of organizing a company, corporation, or business but that organization is contingent on a number of factors; so what works in one organization may not work in another. Some common contingency factors include the organization size, resources, technology, adaptation to the environment, operations activities, motivating forces, staff education, and managerial assumptions. Contingency theory states that the organization must be designed in such a manner as to fit into the environment. Management should utilize the best approach to achieve tasks. Fielder concluded that leadership should be appropriate for the organizational needs and different organizations require different styles of leadership depending upon contingent factors, such as staff, tasks, and other group variables. Vroom and Yetton concluded that success in decision making is contingent on a number of factors, including information available, acceptance of the decision, agreement or disagreement, and the importance of the decision.

CRISIS THEORY

Crisis theory describes how patients respond to crisis situations that interrupt their current practices of self-care. For patients struggling with chronic disease, the crisis may be critical at the time of diagnosis. Individuals may have difficulty coping with their diagnoses because of worry about long-term outcomes or management of daily activities. As patients adjust to living with their chronic disease, for example, the crisis state may be modified and not quite as novel. However, living with chronic disease can always produce new complications, each of which may lead to other situations that disrupt patients' regular habits of managing their self-care.

CHAOS THEORY

Chaos theory was first developed by Denise F. Coppa, as a reflection of the order that is still present within disorganization. The theory states that even within the most disorganized situations, there is still some sense of order. Although change occurs in nursing situations and changes that are very unpredictable can lead to chaos, appropriate management of change can prevent chaos from completely erupting. Nursing involves acceptance of the fact that change is inevitable, and it is more important to learn how to manage change than to try to prevent it. Nurses who understand that not all change is predictable can better respond to changes as they happen. If they can control their response to change, they can prevent it from becoming chaotic.

SOCIAL COGNITIVE THEORY

In the 1970s, A. Bandura proposed the **social cognitive theory,** in which learning develops from observation, and organizing and rehearsing behavior that has been modeled. Bandura believed that people were more likely to adopt the behavior if they valued the outcomes and the outcomes had functional value. He also believed people were more likely to adopt the behavior if the person modeling had similarities to the learner and was admired because of status. Behavior is the result of observation of behavioral, environmental, and cognitive interactions. There are 4 conditions required for modeling:

- **Attention**: The degree of attention paid to modeling can depend on many variables (physical, social, environmental).
- **Retention**: People's ability to retain models depends on symbolic coding, creating mental images, organizing thoughts, and rehearsing (mentally or physically).
- **Reproduction**: The ability to reproduce a model depends on physical and mental capabilities.
- **Motivation**: Motivation may derive from past performances, rewards, or vicarious modeling.

EFFECTS OF SOCIAL COGNITIVE THEORY ON CHANGES IN BEHAVIOR FOR HEALTHY LIFESTYLES

Social cognitive theory was developed by Albert Bandura, who stated that changes are influenced by several factors associated with personal thought and exposure to the environment. When considering healthy lifestyles, social cognitive theory would assess the behavior of others through observation, in that patients could observe others making healthy choices and consider these choices for themselves. The theory also accounts for self-efficacy, which is the belief in the self to be able to do something. Patients making choices for a healthier lifestyle must develop enough self-efficacy to believe that change is possible and that they are able to make appropriate changes. Social cognitive theory also promotes outcome expectancy, which is a belief in the success of the behavior change. To be successful for making healthy lifestyle decisions, patients must believe that the outcomes will be positive.

HEALTH BELIEF MODEL

The **Health Belief Model** was first recognized in the 1950s as a response to the question of why more people did not take measures to maintain their health and prevent disease. The Health Belief Model considers a person's understanding of potential illness and its severity, the patient's risk of contracting the illness, the benefits that would occur if steps were taken to prevent the illness, and potential barriers to prevention measures. The Health Belief Model addresses patients' ideas about health and susceptibility to disease and determines what measures may affect their understanding of illness and prevention. For example, nurses may work with patients at risk for developing diabetes but who do not understand the severity of the complications associated with it. Nurses' roles are to assess the patients' views of the severity of diabetes, their ideas of how susceptible they are to developing it, and their capacity for prevention.

ECOLOGICAL MODEL

The **ecological model** focuses on the interactions between people and their environments (physical, socioeconomic). This model recognizes that behavior reflects multiple levels of influence (intrapersonal, interpersonal, socioeconomic, psychological organizational, community, public policy) and that reciprocal causation (people influence and are influenced by the environment) occurs. Each level of influence may change how a person behaves related to health care. For example, a person may be motivated (intrapersonal factor) to lose weight, but family (interpersonal factor) may resist preparing low calorie meals, and low income (socioeconomic factor) may force the person to buy foods high in simple carbohydrates. In order for health promotion to be effective, environments must be aligned toward the goal because, if they are not, results may be short-lived. However, if the individual lacks motivation or is not interested in changing behavior, supportive environments may be ineffective. It's important to try to align the individual and the environmental factors.

THEORY OF REASONED ACTION

The **Theory of Reasoned Action**, developed in 1975 by Fishbein and Ajzen, is based on the idea that the actions people take voluntarily can be predicted according to their personal attitude toward the action and their perception of how others will view their doing the action. There are 3 basic concepts to the theory:

- **Attitudes:** These are all of the attitudes about an action, and they may be weighted (some more important than others).
- **Subjective norms:** People are influenced by those in their social realm (family, friends) and their attitudes toward particular actions. The influence may be weighted. For example, the attitude of a spouse may carry more weight than the attitude of a neighbor.
- **Behavioral intention:** The intention to take action is based on weighing attitudes and subjective norms (opinions of others), resulting in a choice to either take an action or avoid the action.

Patient-Care Models

CARE MODELS

Depending on the health care unit, various **patient-care models** may be implemented. These models often provide the best patient care available, using methods that meet the needs of specific populations.

- The **team nursing approach** involves a group of nurses where one acts as a team leader. Each team member is responsible for certain types of care, such as medications or activities of daily living. Team nursing may involve a mix of skill levels.
- **Primary nursing** focuses on continuity of care insofar as the same nurse is assigned to care for the same patient over time. This allows the nurse to become very knowledgeable about the patient's needs and provides the patient with a sense of continuity.
- **Total patient care** occurs when the nurse is responsible for all aspects of patient care; this model may also be referred to as case-method nursing.

DECENTRALIZATION

Many nursing units follow similar standards for employees and managers, which often include staff nurses who work in the clinical setting and who are governed by managers who make decisions, uphold standards, and support the mission of the organization. A **decentralized unit** integrates management into the work of the staff, so that instead of one central manager, the work is spread out through the work staff, clinical nurse leaders, and managers. This decentralized concept puts managers within the clinical settings and at the front lines, so that nurses working in clinical units on a day-to-day basis are also the ones making the decisions. Decentralization helps nursing staff to feel more empowered, and decisions are made in the context of clinical situations, which may be more applicable. Decentralization gets more nurses involved in leadership, allowing for participation, pursuit of interest, and retention of information.

SHARED GOVERNANCE MODEL

Shared governance is a process that gives nursing staff the power and ability to work together to make decisions for the unit. While a clinical unit is still managed by one or more leaders, shared governance within the unit establishes roles for staff nurses that support the clinical work and maintain a positive work environment for everyone. Shared governance may involve council work, in that specific councils are established that are composed of teams who work toward a common goal. Each team is made up of staff nurses who work together to promote and support their council activities. Examples of councils might be quality-improvement councils, which seek to educate and establish standards for quality improvement on the clinical unit; an education council, which monitors the educational requirements for staff and provides educational opportunities; or a management council, which performs scheduling, hiring of new staff, and management of issues related to the clinical unit.

MORAL COURAGE

Moral courage involves acting in the best interests of a given situation, even if there are potentially negative consequences as a result. Organizations that support moral courage among their nursing staff may have several similar attributes. They often have developed mission statements that support their vision to uphold ethical patient care. Some organizations may also describe having core values that are essential to their practice and which promote morality or ethical care standards. Health care centers may have nursing practice models in place that describe how nurses work together for patient care; communicate between health providers; and provide safe, effective, and ethical care. A final component is the concept of shared governance among nursing staff. This

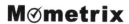

allows staff to make more decisions for themselves, providing greater empowerment when nurses know that they can take steps to support moral courage through their direct patient-care measures.

PARTICIPATIVE MANAGEMENT

Participative management is a style of organization that promotes management of issues at all staff levels. Instead of employing managers who are out of the clinical environment and, therefore, have less knowledge of clinical realities, participatory management considers the input of nurses at all levels, from bedside staff nurses to clinical nurse leaders to nursing supervisors. Nurses assist each other by providing skills or imparting knowledge of situations in which they have expertise or have encountered previously. In this way, ideas are shared, and all nurses have access to communication, knowledge, and guidance among themselves to ensure appropriate patient care while instilling the values and expertise to everyone in the unit.

SYNERGISTIC MODEL

Synergy occurs between nurses and patients when both parties work together for patient care, using methods that support and enhance the actions of the other. When nursing care is synergistic with that of patients, optimal outcomes occur. All individuals in the model have their own responsibilities toward working together. Nurses provide patient care and education that are sensitive to patients' needs; nurses involve the patient's families when appropriate, allowing patients to take part in decision-making for their care; and nurses display competence in their actions. Patients' roles in the synergistic model are to participate in health decisions regarding their care, receive education and instruction from nurses, follow measures for treatment and prevention, and recognize the competence of nurses.

OMAHA SYSTEM OF TAXONOMY

The **Omaha System** was developed by a group of nurses in Omaha, Nebraska, in 1975 and was adopted by the American Nurses Association in 1992. It is used to measure patient outcomes, describe nursing interventions, and document patient needs. The system is made up of three parts. The problem classification uses information gained from assessments of patients and how they are affected by the environment, health-related behaviors, physiological effects, and psychosocial aspects. The intervention scheme guides nurses in developing nursing interventions for patients' conditions, as seen by the problem classification. The intervention scheme consists of several categories, including guidance of patients, surveillance, treatments of patients, and case management. The third scheme consists of a scale for rating the patients' problems, which can help to evaluate overall progress. This scheme is further broken down to analyze patients' knowledge, behavior, and health status.

LEVINE'S CONSERVATION MODEL

Myra Levine was a nurse who developed the **Conservation Model** that considers each nurse–patient relationship as an individual connection by adapting holistic approaches, such as the person, the environment, the patient's adaptation, and the patient's response as a person. Conservation is defined as keeping a patient in a state of wholeness or integrity when normal coping abilities are disturbed. The components of the model are to promote patient adaptation and to support wholeness of the patient as a person, to help the nurse understand the patient's responses to care (e.g., behavioral changes, stress, patient perception), and to maintain the principles of integrity by conserving energy and maintaining the structure of the process.

MEDICAL MODEL VS. PATIENT-CENTERED MODEL OF CARE

The patient-centered model of care can differ from the medical model insofar as patients play a distinct role in making decisions about their own care.

- Within the **medical model**, clinicians may develop a paternalistic view of patient care, in which they tell patients what they need to do for treatment without offering patients a chance for further input. The medical model often focuses on the diseases or illnesses that are present and seeks to find methods of treatment, with which patients may or may not agree.
- Alternatively, the **patient-centered model** allows patients to have a say in the care they receive. They participate in the decision-making process for their treatment goals. Care is focused on quality of life for patients, rather than focusing primarily on disease. The patient-centered model allows patients and physicians to work together to devise goals that will most clearly benefit patients.

PATIENT-CENTERED CARE

Patients are often hospitalized under circumstances that are frightening or confusing; the care environment often adds to these feelings when physicians and staff talk in jargon, patients are not aware of the timing of their treatments or medications, and nurses do not give patients the respect they are due. Nurses can improve the clinical areas where they work to make the environment more patient-friendly, which improves patient-centered care practices. Nurses can help to make patients and their families comfortable in the hospital environment by being available to answer questions as needed, providing privacy and quiet when patients wish, answering call lights quickly, accommodating family or visitors when appropriate, and staying with patients during treatments or procedures.

CONCEPT OF CARING

Caring involves feeling compassion for people and helping them to do things that they may not be able to do themselves. Within nursing, caring requires knowledge of the skills used to provide caring measures. When establishing a patient-centered environment, nurses must consider caring a form of attention that centers around what patients truly need. Many patients have difficulty being hospitalized or receiving medical treatment. They may feel unsure about their diagnoses, anxious finances, or isolated in their condition. Nurses who provide care meet patients at these levels, easing some of their anxiety, providing education to meet learning needs, or counteracting loneliness. These strategies and many others are at the core of patient-centered care because they are directed at patients and are designed to provide holistic and therapeutic interventions.

CLINICAL MICROSYSTEM

A **clinical microsystem** is a particular setting of clinical care that uses a specific group of people to provide care for patients. Those providing care in the microsystem work together to care for patients on a regular basis, and many patients who receive care fall into a certain population who are most likely to need care in this setting. Microsystems contain essential elements to their functioning, including patients who receive services, nursing and support staff who are trained to work in these settings, processes of care that have been designed to meet the care of the specific patient populations, and an information system developed to track and record the care given in this setting.

SUCCESSFUL HEALTH CARE MICROSYSTEMS

Successful microsystems provide patient care to specific populations in a timely and organized manner that meets patients' needs. There are several characteristics that are common among successful microsystems, including quality leadership, patient-focused care, educated and trained staff, organizational support, and community support. Those who provide leadership in the microsystem help the group to achieve shared goals while acting as resources for staff and patients. Patient-focused care concentrates on meeting patients' needs through sensitive care, education, quick responses, and timely direction. Nurses who are well educated and trained in their specific job functions understand the best methods of care delivery and implement high standards into practice. Often, microsystems are associated with larger organizations, whose support is vital to maintaining a solid and successful program. Finally, the support of the community drives patients to seek care within the specific microsystem and keeps them coming back.

Interprofessional Team

INTERDISCIPLINARY TEAM APPROACH

The **interdisciplinary team approach** involves various disciplines working together as a team to provide comprehensive care for patients. Specific patients may need several disciplines to work together to manage their care in addition to nursing and medicine, such as social services, mental health, occupational or physical therapy, or spiritual care. The interdisciplinary team model differs from the multidisciplinary approach that also uses several disciplines to provide patient care; for example, while the multidisciplinary approach involves using several disciplines, practitioners typically work on their own and provide information as needed; additionally, the practitioners are often limited to one or more visits. The interdisciplinary team approach involves meeting together and collaborating to develop appropriate outcomes that are in the patient's best interest. Team members coordinate their efforts throughout the patient's stay.

DEVELOPING A CARE PLAN

Developing a patient care plan involves using whichever disciplines are necessary for the patients' specific needs to reach their health care goals. The process of developing a care plan as part of an interdisciplinary team first involves assessing the various needs of patients throughout several disciplines. For example, a patient may require services from a physician, nutritionist, and occupational therapist in addition to standard nursing care. Once the disciplines have been identified, the team meets to develop the plan of care, using services to list interventions and develop outcomes. After devised practices have been implemented, the team later evaluates the effectiveness of interventions and revises goals as necessary.

CLINICAL NURSE LEADERS AS RESOURCES

Clinical nurse leaders are unit-specific roles in that each nurse leader is employed to work directly with certain units and populations of patients. Each role is set within certain microsystems that are embedded within health care facilities, outpatient clinics, or stand-alone centers. Because the role is unit-specific, clinical nurse leaders are experts in the care of the specific populations of patients that they serve. Clinical nurse leaders have access to various types of resources within the community, the health care organization, and professional groups targeted toward care within their specific microsystem. Clinical nurse leaders can help staff to meet their patient-care goals by providing assistance with direct care, helping solve problems that may occur, communicating with health care providers and other members of the interdisciplinary team, or working with management to bring attention to current issues or shortcomings that may need to be changed.

NURSES' NURSE

Clinical nurse leaders are not only present to help bridge communication between practitioners and to coordinate care, but part of their role is to work with nursing staff to support their work. Clinical nurse leaders may be referred to as the **"nurses' nurse,"** as they often act as a nurse for the nursing staff by coordinating efforts and assisting staff nurses in some of their work. Clinical nurse leaders may provide nursing care in times of staff shortages or for particularly busy units. Part of this role may also involve working with clinical preceptors who train new staff to develop appropriate instructional materials. Clinical nurse leaders may also act as mentors to staff by being the point of contact for nurses when they need guidance, assistance, or educational services.

CHAIN OF COMMAND

USING CHAIN OF COMMAND TO PROVIDE APPROPRIATE PATIENT CARE

The **chain of command** is the order of authority for health care decision-making among providers. Orders may be passed along the chain of command; alternatively, when nurses are in a position where they do not know how to respond, they may use the chain of command to ask for help. To use the chain of command appropriately, staff nurses first contact their supervising nurse or the charge nurse. If the charge nurse cannot or does not help, nurses may then ask for help from the director or supervisor of the unit. The chief nursing officer is above the nursing director and is ultimately above all nurses in the organization. The chief nursing officer is the head authority for decision-making and can be contacted as part of seeking guidance when other attempts at advocacy among nursing managers or supervisors have failed.

DECIDING NOT TO USE THE CHAIN OF COMMAND TO SEEK HELP FOR WORK

The chain of command is designed to protect nurses, their patients, and organizations as a whole. Nurses who use the chain of command seek help in making decisions about what to do next or how to handle certain difficult situations. There may be times, however, when nurses do not use the chain of command. Some nurses do not like to ask for help because they do not want to appear incompetent. There may be some nurses who do not believe they need help or who think that they have enough information or knowledge to handle the situation. Some nurses do not seek help because they do not necessarily care about the outcomes of the situations with which they are dealing, which could put them at risk of harming patients or put the organization at risk for legal issues. Finally, some nurses do not use the chain of command because they do not know to whom to turn when they need help.

CRITICAL THINKING

Critical thinking is a process that reflects on the work of nurses, the status of patients, and the environment of care to determine the next action to be tackled. Nursing requires critical thinking skills to provide care and treatment successfully, reduce risks for patients, and improve the overall quality of the health care environment. Nurses use critical thinking skills before making decisions to pursue interventions. They base these decisions on the nursing diagnoses for the patients and their current conditions, considering what impact the interventions will have on patients. Nurses must be familiar with the nursing process as well as the specific interventions they will employ to help them discern what results might occur. Following the implementation of interventions, nurses then use critical thinking to evaluate the effectiveness of their actions to determine whether practice changes need to be made.

TRAITS FOR CRITICAL THINKING

The nurse who uses critical thinking skills possesses certain **intellectual traits** that make critical thinking successful.

- **Intellectual humility** is the ability of the nurse to admit that she does not know something about a particular situation. The nurse is willing to accept the advice or direction of another person who has more knowledge than she does.

- **Intellectual integrity** occurs when the nurse continues to evaluate her own thoughts and ideas about the situations she encounters. Part of the process of intellectual integrity is when the nurse admits her willingness to see others' viewpoints or admit a wrong.
- Finally, **intellectual empathy** happens when the nurse puts aside her own opinions or judgments for the sake of providing consistent care. This involves empathizing with others and being willing to consider their feelings and how it would be to walk in their place.

PROBLEM SOLVING

Nurses must use their critical thinking skills to **solve problems** that they may encounter in their work. Once the problem is earmarked, nurses must identify potential resources or information that will help them to understand the scope of the problem. Next, nurses must develop possible solutions for solving the problem. They then evaluate all possible solutions, determining the positive and negative aspects of each, as well as potential consequences of selection. Nurses then must choose one of the solutions as their choice for solving the problem and implementing it into practice. Finally, nurses must evaluate the success of their decisions by determining how well their interventions are solving the problem.

Patient Advocacy

KEY HEALTH CARE DISPARITIES

Health care disparities are those factors that increase risk to one population over other populations related to health. Disparities may include:

- **Socioeconomic status**: Includes employment, income level, debts, support systems. Those with inadequate income may not be able to afford adequate health care or pay for treatment. Some may experience discrimination and increased stress, affecting health.
- **Environment**: Includes housing issues, available transportation, access to parks, walkways, and geography. Those who are homeless or lack transportation, for example, may not be able to access health care.
- **Education**: Those who have inadequate health literacy may have poor understanding of health concerns and neglect conditions that require treatment or fail to follow through with treatments.
- **Diet/Food**: Some may lack access to healthy foods or go hungry, affecting health.
- **System:** Includes insurance coverage, quality of health care, availability of providers, and cultural competency of providers.
- **Ethnicity:** Some groups have higher risks for certain diseases, such as African Americans and hypertension.

PATIENTS' DECISION-MAKING
BEING AN ADVOCATE FOR DECISION-MAKING BY PATIENTS

The nurse plays a critical role in assisting patients with making decisions about their care. Patients who are informed and involved in their care decisions may have high quality of care, improved outcomes, and may feel more empowered about their own health. Nurses act as **advocates** for their patients' decision-making by ensuring that patients have adequate information, which is correct for their situations. Nurses ensure that patients have access to appropriate health information by giving them resources, materials, or education through instruction or speaking with the interdisciplinary team. Nurses help patients to determine their own priorities without subjecting them to their own personal beliefs. They then verify their patients' decisions and support them as they make choices about their own care.

PATIENTS' DECISION-MAKING STANDARDS

According to the American Medical Association, there are three main components of **appropriate decision-making on the part of patients**.

- **Clinical information** involves giving patients adequate information to allow them to make decisions about their care. Without adequate information, patients are not informed enough to make appropriate decisions. Nurses must ensure that patients have the information they need to make an informed decision.
- **Clarifying values** takes into consideration what is important to patients in terms of their expectations for outcomes and treatments or management. It shows patients that their needs are recognized and are a pertinent aspect of their care.
- **Guidance** assists patients with making their decisions but also with communicating to others what they have decided.

PATERNALISTIC APPROACH

Patients have a right to make decisions about their own care; the attitudes of nurses who provide information to patients have a big impact on how patients receive the information and make decisions for themselves. **Paternalism** occurs when nurses or physicians give information to the patient, with little or no input from patients about their own desires or decisions. The paternalistic approach often assumes that nurses or physicians know what is best for patients in terms of their health—even more than the patients themselves. The flow of information is one way: from health care providers to patients. Paternalism removes patients' autonomy by not giving them the ability to make informed decisions and instead by seeking to keep them in an inferior position as receivers of care, rather than as informed and knowledgeable participants.

INFORMATION DISCLOSURE

All patients have certain **rights** when seeking medical treatment that are part of the nurse's position to uphold. Information disclosure involves informing patients about the information they need to know when seeking care at a specific health care facility. This information includes data about the facility, such as its accreditation status, procedures for filing complaints, and the center's positions on certain types of treatments, such as life-saving measures. Additionally, information disclosure involves telling patients about the expertise, licensure, and certification status of the health care providers who will be caring for them. Patients are also notified about their rights to receive information in a way that they understand, specifically if they have a disability that may prevent them from comprehending the given information. This includes the right to a language interpreter, a mental health worker, a patient advocate, or any other method of providing information to patients with disabilities.

INFORMED PATIENTS

Patients who are informed about their care and treatment may make better decisions that ultimately impact the overall cost of health care services. Cutting corners by providing less information because of time constraints may lead to miscommunication because of misunderstandings. Patients who do not receive enough information about their health may not follow directions correctly, thus leading to inadequate care or potential failure of the treatment. Inadequate treatments may lead to repeat admissions or improper use of facilities, such as going to the emergency department for situations that are not urgent. Patients who truly understand their medical conditions, that is, how sick they really are or what their prognoses are, may be more likely go to follow up appointments, consultations, or rehabilitation. Patients are also more likely to take their medications as prescribed when they are informed, resulting in fewer medication errors or repeated prescriptions.

27

ADVANCE DIRECTIVES

An **advance directive** is a document signed by patients that explains their wishes for their health care. The advance directive is developed in the event that patients are unable to make decisions for themselves. A living will is a signed and notarized document that is written with the patients' wishes for their treatment, particularly life-saving care in the event that they have a terminal illness. The living will designates terms for withdrawing life support in the event that patients are unable to make their wishes known because of illness. Alternatively, a durable power of attorney exists when patients designate a representative to make health care decisions for them. This document must be signed and notarized to be valid. A durable power of attorney does not require that patients have a terminal condition to be valid, but the designated representatives do have rights to make treatment decisions in the best interests of the patients regardless of their condition.

PROTECTING PATIENTS' RIGHT TO PRIVACY

Patients' right to privacy is valid in any type of health care setting, from the hospital to the long-term care center. There are several measures that nurse leaders can practice in a clinical setting that help patients to understand that their privacy is being protected and they are respected as individuals. When discussing sensitive information, nurses should refrain from talking to patients in front of others. Instead, they should close the door or have the conversation in a private area. Patients should be allowed to undress and be examined in an area that is private and separate from other patients and visitors. When patients stay in the health care center, their rooms should be treated as personal spaces; nurses should knock before entering and maintain the space as private. Finally, nurses should never touch patients' personal items without first asking permission, except in cases of emergency.

PRESERVE THE DIGNITY OF PATIENTS

Patients who seek help for physical or emotional issues need not only treatment and management through nursing care, but they must also receive services in a manner that preserves their dignity and signifies respect. Nurses who care for patients who have mental health issues or experience psychological distress can **protect their patients' dignity** through their actions while providing care. This is done by asking questions to determine how they can help, using positive body language, and using active listening skills. Nurses should try to provide as much information about the situation as possible if it will help to ease distress. Nurses should also consider family members and their responses to the event by including them in discussions of care when appropriate. If necessary, patients may need a referral for counseling to discuss their emotional state and to look for resources for managing their mental health.

VULNERABLE PATIENT POPULATIONS

The CNL must take an active role in **advocating for vulnerable patient populations**:

- **Elderly**: Includes being alert to signs of abuse and neglect and reporting to appropriate authorities, providing information about community resources, assessing for risk factors, such as falls, poor nutrition, vision/hearing impairment, assisting patient to maintain a safe environment (safety bars, elimination of throw rugs, adequate lighting), and providing information about advance directives and end-of-life planning.
- **Low health literacy**: Includes assessing literacy and providing appropriate materials and education, ensuring that patients are aware of resources available to them, understand how to access those resources, and understand their rights and responsibilities as patients.

- **Low socioeconomic status**: Includes assessing mental, physical, and social status, determining needs, providing information/education, and assisting the person to access resources (free clinics, low-cost health care providers, Medicaid, food banks, homeless shelters, low-cost housing, various community resources, faith-based programs, 12-step programs, mental-health programs, support groups).

PATIENT ADVOCACY BEYOND BEDSIDE NURSING CARE

Patient advocacy extends **beyond care given at the bedside**. Nurses may act as patient advocates by speaking in the community at various levels. Advocacy for patient care may be in the form of contacting organizations to find support for patient care. It may involve working with health care administrators to change policies and procedures that reflect evidence-based practices for best patient care. Some nurses write editorials or letters to authority figures, using their medical knowledge to back up their opinions. Other nurses may contact politicians, volunteer in grassroots organizations, speak at conferences or on public forums, or testify before legislatures.

KEY STAKEHOLDERS WHEN ADVOCATING FOR HEALTH CARE CHANGES

Engaging stakeholders, those with a vested interested in evidence-based practice, is critical when advocating for health care changes. Stakeholders may include:

- **Patients and their families, caregivers, and advocates**: Information should be tied to personal interests so people understand benefits and presented in a manner that is understandable to the lay person, avoiding medical jargon or complex data.
- **Health care providers**: Clinicians need clear evidence of benefit to themselves and patients with supporting data.
- **Health care organizations and associations**: Emphasis should include benefits to the organization in terms of reduced error or improved patient care as well as cost-effectiveness and return-on-investment.
- **Employers and insurers**: The explanation for the need of coverage for any changes in practice should be clearly outlined, including data regarding benefits, such as reduced hospital stay or reduced complications.
- **Health care industry/Manufacturers**: These may have product information that can be very helpful as part of implementation.
- **Policymakers**: Providing the most up-to-date information in a format that is easy to understand and supported by adequate data can help with decision-making.

BARRIERS TO EFFECTIVE PATIENT ADVOCACY

Patient advocacy is a key component of what nurses do in their everyday work. Advocacy involves speaking on behalf of their patients to fulfill their needs, particularly when they cannot speak for themselves. Although this is a pertinent role of nurses, there are some **barriers to effective advocacy.** Some nurses do not believe that they can make a difference, and so they fail to speak up. They believe that no one will listen, and they do not want to waste their time. There are some nurses who do not know where to go to be heard, whether it is following the chain of command or speaking in other situations outside of direct patient care. Some nurses think that advocacy takes too much time. Finally, some nurses feel that if they speak up as advocates, they may face negative consequences or feedback where they work.

EDUCATING PATIENTS ABOUT THEIR CHRONIC DISEASE

Providing education about **chronic conditions** is challenging enough due to diminished health literacy as well as financial implications surrounding disease management. Patients who suffer from chronic diseases in which there are few symptoms or symptoms come and go may be less likely to listen to nursing education or continue with follow-up care. For example, patients diagnosed with heart disease may have hypertension or high cholesterol, both of which may result in few symptoms despite being illnesses that require consistent monitoring and lifestyle changes. Nurses who provide teaching about these illnesses may have patients who do not want to follow through with orders because they may not be suffering physical symptoms. Additionally, nurses may have challenges with patients who manage symptoms that resolve. Despite the fact that symptoms have abated, nurses must continue to provide ongoing education.

BARRIERS FACED WHEN ACCESSING HEALTH CARE

Patients may face many different types of barriers when attempting to **access care** for their health. Nurse leaders should recognize these barriers as a first attempt at addressing issues related to health care access for patient populations. Geographic barriers are those that arise when patients are unable to access care because of where they live. It may be difficult for them to get to appointments or to reach the nearest health care organization to receive adequate health services. Financial barriers exist when patients are unable to pay for the services they need. They may not have health insurance or may be denied insurance for certain procedures. Cultural barriers exist when patients disagree with practices performed by health care providers, such that they do not want to follow orders or follow through with treatments. In some cases, cultural barriers also cause misunderstandings so that patients do not know what they are supposed to do to follow through with treatments or to attend appointments.

Nursing Advocacy

ADVOCACY FOR THE NURSING PROFESSION

Advocacy is the process of defending or speaking up for people, often when they cannot speak for themselves. There is a lot of literature about the role of nurses as advocates for their patients, but clinical nurse leaders must also act as advocates for the nursing profession. Nurse leaders are in a unique position to work with various disciplines and skill levels, to offer insight, and to lend support for the nursing profession as an essential career. Clinical nurse leaders may work with patients, other nurses, administrators, physicians, and with various disciplines on teams. Through these interactions, they can educate others about the importance of nursing, communicate with others about the distinct role nurses play in the interdisciplinary team, and advocate for the rights of working nurses to be decision-makers. Among nursing staff, clinical nurse leaders may advocate for the profession by supporting other nurses, providing guidance in decisions, and invoking a sense of teamwork that encourages feelings of pride.

PROFESSIONAL PRACTICE ADVOCACY

Professional practice advocacy is the process of advocating for the nursing profession as a valid and ever-changing profession. Advocacy may involve supporting the rights of nurses as professionals in both their places of employment or within the educational system. The practice of nursing may need to be defended against administrators, insurance companies, or legislators, all of whom may be striving to make cuts in employment or salaries or simply do not understand the complexities of nursing roles. Nurses may advocate for their profession by speaking with legislators, political officials, and the public to educate them about the essential roles within the profession. They may join organizations or start a group of their own to act as a voice for nursing support. Nurses also support the profession by promoting change in the health care environment, such as by changing policies, supporting flexible scheduling and pay increases, and encouraging employee health and wellness.

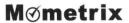

PROMOTING ADVANCEMENT IN EDUCATION

Nurse leaders have opportunities to **endorse the benefits of pursuing an advanced degree** in nursing among the nurses with whom they work by acting on their own roles as nurses with advanced educations. Many nurses receive the minimum amount of training required to practice in the clinical environment without pursuing higher educational degrees. Nurse leaders can encourage other nurses to pursue advanced education by promoting learning throughout clinical work through teaching, educational seminars, or detailed instruction; reminding nurses that an advanced degree may lead to more professional opportunities and higher pay; showing nurses some of the ways to advance their degrees, such as through online programs or evening classes; or acting as character references for nurses who wish to pursue advanced training.

ADVOCATING FOR EXPANDED EDUCATION OF STAFF

Clinical nurse leaders act as **advocates to advance the education of the staff** with whom they work. Clinical nurse leaders participate in leadership and decision-making and model this behavior with their colleagues. Clinical nurse leaders that have a master's degree set an example for others about what advanced educational experiences mean; they may also work with nursing instructors who are developing practical experiences for students in nursing programs, or they may act as preceptors to help train students or new staff. Within their role, clinical nurse leaders may also provide educational opportunities for others by acting as teachers or presenters of information that is pertinent to patient care standards within their field of expertise.

AUTONOMY

Much nursing literature is devoted to the **autonomy** of patients or control over their own care; however, nurses have a right to expect autonomy in their own care environments. Within the nursing role, autonomy involves control over making decisions for patient care, as well as for other aspects of employment, such as work schedules or staffing. Most staff nurses do not want someone outside the organization or the unit to make decisions for them regarding these activities, but instead want to play an active role in deciding and acting on situations that fall within their scope of practice. Although nurses are still accountable for their decisions, improving nursing autonomy allows nurses to feel competent, satisfied, and committed to their work.

INFLUENCE

Influence is the ability of nurses to convince others with a different set of beliefs of their position. When approaching decision-makers, nurses should first develop a plan of action regarding their goals for new decisions. They should identify how they will approach leaders and know with whom to talk. Nurses can better influence others of their agenda if they have confidence in themselves, their background, and their knowledge of the subject. It is important to use influence enough so that it can change the minds of the appropriate people without coming across as too pushy. Too much effort at convincing others through argument or debate may lead to tension and defensiveness.

POWER

Power is the ability to control or exert influence in a given situation. Nurses can be powerful because of their knowledge and expertise in caring for patients to influence legislation for changes in health policies.

- **Expert power** comes from having the knowledge and skill within a certain area to be credible enough to speak about certain issues. Nurses can use their expert power to describe how changes in health policies impact patient care.

31

- **Legitimate power** comes from having a certain status. Nurses are trained and educated in patient care and, therefore, have legitimate power because of their position to influence the legislative environment.
- **Referent power** comes from having the respect of others. Nursing is a respected profession for its caring provision, knowledge and skill in practice and, as such, can be a powerful force to influence decisions that impact health care.

HEALTH POLICY PLANNING AND CHANGE

Although health care continues to require policy development and changes in practice, many professionals, such as government officials, insurance companies, and physicians are those who are actually practicing to make changes. However, because nurses are people who are most involved in patient care, they should be the ones backing policy changes. Because nurses provide patient care, education, quality improvement, and research studies in the clinical environment, they are the ones who are often the most knowledgeable about areas in need of change. Nurses serve as powerful **advocates for change** in many areas, including preventive measures, wellness initiatives, cost reductions, patient safety, reduction of medical errors, and reduction of fraud and abuse. Not only are nurses knowledgeable about health care needs, but they are also compassionate and giving as a group. These factors, when combined, make nurses a force for change that needs to be encouraged in the social and political arenas to support policy development, research initiatives, and funding.

INFLUENCING HEALTH LEGISLATION

Nurses may often feel that they have little power when it comes to **influencing legislation** to make changes in health policies, but nurses are actually the ideal candidates to inspire change in this area. Many nurses do not know what to do to get involved with legislation, but by working with mentors or other advocates, more nurses can learn the process and become competent about legislation. Some professional organizations offer workshops, conferences, or educational classes that provide information about the process and allow nurses to meet others who are also trying to make changes. Nurses may support change by writing letters to representatives, calling elected officials, or attending public meetings that address health issues. They may also speak to groups to discuss proposed issues or work with the media to increase attention to their causes.

IMPACTING HEALTH POLICY REFORM

Nurses can make an impact on health policy to make themselves heard about changes that need to be made in the health care system. A nurse can take action on several levels to influence **health policy reform**.

- At the **institutional level**, nurses may serve on committees or lobby the organization's administration to make changes in policies and procedures in the hospital or clinic where they work.
- At the **community level**, nurses may speak with community leaders, promote outcomes through evidence-based practice by working with nursing organizations, or establish health policies in public health and preventive care.
- At the **national level**, nurses may work with legislators and politicians to educate them about the importance of certain health standards, speak to groups about health policy reform, or serve on national committees for nursing organizations to shape policy changes within the group.

LOBBYING

Lobbying is defined as trying to influence politicians or people in power to make legislative changes on certain issues. Nurses can be effective lobbyists by knowing the issues about which they speak; being credible about their background and their work performance; networking with others to find help backing their positions, particularly with those in office or those with political influence; understanding their opponents who speak against their issues; directly asking for what they want from legislators and policy makers; and being willing to work at all lobbying levels, including the organizational level, the community level, and the national level.

WHISTLEBLOWERS

Whistleblowers are people who recognize a form of wrongdoing where they work and who report the situation so that it can be corrected or otherwise rectified. There are laws in place that protect nurses who become whistleblowers from being penalized by their employers for their actions, although there are still some nurses who choose to look the other way in the face of illegal activity. Some reasons why nurses may not want to report a violation are that they feel uncomfortable with the situation and do not know to whom to report. Nurses may have moral or ethical dilemmas themselves with the situation, which may cause confusion about what to report and why. Although nurses may technically not face legal retaliation about reporting fraud or illegal practices, they may still face scrutiny and harassment from their employers and coworkers, which may make them afraid to do the right thing.

PROFESSIONAL PRESENTATIONS

Nurse leaders may have opportunities to present information about their clinical practices during seminars or conferences. These **presentations** are often designed for discussions that affect nurses or other health professionals. By presenting information, nurses disseminate their knowledge of the subject to inform and educate others for their own practices. They may use slide show presentations to present graphs and charts and discuss the data. A slide show presentation is ideal when nurses need to present a large amount of information. Another option is a poster presentation, which consists of one large display with all the information up front. This may be an option for small projects that have fewer data. Writing an article or an abstract is another way to present information. An abstract contains all of the essential data that nurses wish to present, but abstracts must be submitted and accepted for publication.

DISSEMINATING CLINICAL INFORMATION

There may be times when nurses have opportunities to share their clinical experiences with other professionals or with members of other disciplines in venues outside of their immediate clinical practice unit. Such times are often opportunities for networking and growth for nurses through educational or professional settings. Nurses may serve on a panel for discussion, in which they and other experts answer questions about their clinical experiences and practice. They may also present information through the media, including interviews or videos where they describe their work. Nurses may also have opportunities to disseminate information about their patient care by writing pieces for scholarly journals, nursing websites, or professional newsletters.

Professional Identity of the Clinical Nurse Leader

CLINICAL NURSE LEADERS

Clinical nurse leaders make a great impact on quality of health care, and their presence may help relieve some pitfalls associated with current nursing shortages in clinical care. Clinical nurse leaders provide direction, guidance, and support for clinical activities within specific microsystems where they have expertise. They use evidence-based practices to make changes in policies and care standards, which improve patient care practices. They provide supervisory support for staff nurses; this helps with clinical decision-making and relieves some pressure from staff nurses by having support through collaboration. Clinical nurse leaders also eliminate fragmentation in care, providing a smooth stay for patients. Health care centers that employ clinical nurse leaders may see improvements in several areas of patient care, including a reduction in patient injuries and infections, decreased staff nurse turnover, greater satisfaction of patients with hospitalizations, and fewer readmissions after dismissal.

NEED FOR MORE CLINICAL NURSE LEADERS

The profession of nursing is currently facing several critical issues that will take time, energy, financial support, and increased advocacy to overcome. The **need for clinical nurse leaders** is greater now than ever before. While many students pursue nursing as a career and meet the nursing shortage, these students often go through associate-level programs, rather than pursuing a bachelor's degree. While these programs educate students about clinical needs, they may fall short in other areas of education, such as critical thinking or advanced leadership skills. Alternatively, nursing care is very specialized, and nurses continue to perform well beyond the traditional scope of practice of only a few years ago. In addition, some hospitals offer low-quality care because of nursing shortages. All of these issues point to the need for clinical nurse leaders in the health care environment.

EDUCATIONAL REQUIREMENTS

Clinical nurse leaders play a role that is somewhat similar to clinical nurse specialists (CNSs); however, clinical nurse leaders have less **educational preparation** than CNSs. Currently, CNSs are considered advanced-practice registered nurses; however, the role of a clinical nurse leader does require a master's degree in nursing. Clinical nurse specialists may act as resources for clinical nurse leaders when issues arise that are difficult to solve without further leadership intervention. In practice, clinical nurse leaders and clinical nurse specialists' work together to strengthen the units where they work by communicating with staff nurses, providing education, and reviewing evidence-based practices that may need implementation.

EDUCATION MODELS

Clinical nurse leaders must have a master's degree; however, there may be several **avenues** by which to achieve this level of education, depending on the background education of the nurse. A nurse who has a bachelor's degree in nursing may pursue a master's degree program designed for students with a nursing background; however, students who do not have a background in nursing may pursue a master's degree as a second-degree program, which covers more nursing information for the clinical nurse leader. There are also completion track programs for nurses who have only completed an associate's degree or a diploma program before they apply to a master's program. The completion track is designed to fill in the gaps of information found in both associate's degree and diploma programs to allow the nurse to graduate with a master's degree in a short amount of time.

MASTER'S LEVEL EDUCATION

A **master's level education** provides extended opportunities for study and for practice that further prepare clinical nurse leaders for their eventual roles. Ultimately, a master's degree in nursing prepares clinical nurse leaders in developing quality-improvement plans and educating others to carry them out, performing research to determine better methods of practice, building teams of professionals and leading others in their skills and capacities for care, writing new policies or changing existing policies to meet patients' needs, and providing education to other nurses to support continuing education. While many nurses serve in some of these capacities, a master's degree educates graduates more specifically in their roles, beyond the scope of a bachelor's degree program in nursing.

LICENSURE AND CERTIFICATION

While maintaining a valid nursing **license** is a requirement of practice, having a license also establishes credibility with patients and families. The fact that nurses completed training requirements and then passed the necessary tests to gain licensure demonstrates competency. Because licensure requires continuing education, patients and their families know that nurses who have kept their license for many years have continued competence and have continued to maintain their skills and knowledge.

Certification goes beyond licensure and is often specialized for particular areas. Certification often involves proof of practice as well as a testing process so nurses can demonstrate their expertise. Nurses who are certified in their specialty give the message to others that they are professionals with abundant knowledge and background education in their field.

Capacity of the CNL Practice

ROLE OF CLINICAL NURSE LEADERS

The **role of clinical nurse leaders** was developed in response to several issues affecting the health care system. Health care organizations have been faced with nursing shortages, poor-quality patient outcomes, and negative work environments. The role of clinical nurse leaders was developed to take action against some of these critical situations. Clinical nurse leaders take on the responsibilities of assisting with clinical nursing tasks, analyzing quality outcomes, and implementing changes in the work environment and in methods of patient care. The clinical nurse leader specialty was implemented into practice in 2007.

CLINICAL NURSE LEADERS AS EDUCATORS

Education is an essential component of the clinical nurse leaders' job. Nurse leaders **provide education** for colleagues, patients, and the community. When working with patients, nurse leaders support the education given by the bedside nurse to uphold continuity and to reinforce pertinent ideas. Clinical nurse leaders may also provide education to patients through separate instruction, patient groups, or by meeting with patients and their families to provide individualized education. They may also work with community members by offering classes or forums that allow others to learn important health information. Nurse leaders may contact physicians' offices or clinics to partner with them in bringing the public important information. Finally, nurse leaders may promote health education by writing or publishing in journals, newsletters, or other publications available to community members.

POSITION OF CNLs WORKING WITH PATIENTS' FAMILIES

Clinical nurse leaders work with **family members and patients** by meeting with them regularly to determine if their needs are being met or if there are other options for care that should be implemented. Clinical nurse leaders may provide education to families and patients about their specific conditions, surgical procedures, or preventive care. They may also give them information about community resources or social services if extended arrangements need to be made. If patients or their families have concerns or questions about treatments or therapies, clinical nurse leaders may act as liaisons between the family and the physician to foster communication and reduce misunderstandings.

COORDINATORS FOR THE INTERDISCIPLINARY TEAM

Clinical nurse leaders are integral **members of the interdisciplinary team.** Not only do they work with team members to represent nursing services, they may also serve as coordinators for the team, which may mean arranging meetings with team members, organizing information about patients, and keeping track of how team members document on the patients' records. They may also act as liaisons between patients and the rest of the team, for example, by keeping patients informed about when the team meets. If patients do not understand the information discussed in the meeting or if they feel that the team is somehow not hearing them, clinical nurse leaders advocate for patients and provide education to clarify what information was discussed.

MENTORS

Clinical nurse leaders act as **mentors and models** for nurses in the clinical unit. As mentors, clinical nurse leaders work with new staff and provide feedback about their activities, including positive information and areas of concern. They reflect on their practice and discuss their work activities to review the necessary duties for working on the unit. Clinical nurse leaders also teach new staff how to perform certain clinical activities that may be specific to the nursing unit. They may arrange for educational opportunities to provide important information about specific nursing care. The role of clinical nurse leaders as a mentor is ongoing, continuing even after the official training period has ended. They remain resources for all staff as they can help with clinical activities, provide feedback about their work, or guide them in their continued patient care.

QUALITY PATIENT OUTCOMES

By acting as mentors, clinical nurse leaders use their knowledge, educational background, and expertise to train and guide others in their work. This guidance and leadership promote quality outcomes for patients because they improve overall nursing care. When staff nurses or nursing students see a need for change or have questions or comments about their practices, they can approach clinical nurse leaders for guidance about how to proceed. Clinical nurse leaders work with the staff nurses to implement changes as necessary or to evaluate their work and provide constructive feedback. Mentoring and feedback are always designed to improve nursing care, benefitting patients as they receive services.

ROLE MODELS FOR HEALTHY BEHAVIORS

Nurses are **role models for healthy behaviors** whether they want this role or not. A large component of patient care is teaching and education, and the nurses' own behaviors may impact how the message comes across to the patient. For example, nurses who are educating patients about the health risks of smoking should not be seen smoking a cigarette outside the hospital. Most patients would find it difficult to respond to nurses who provide teaching without incorporating the actions that they teach. Although nurses cannot be expected to be perfect in upholding all lifestyle methods that they promote, they should be aware that patients and families are probably using them as role models for their own behaviors.

HEALTH AND WELLNESS COACH

Although there are several disciplines that focus on health and wellness, such as exercise trainers or nutritionists, nurses are in a unique position to provide health and wellness information to patients based on their health expertise. Nurses may provide **health and wellness information** to patients through such measures as teaching patients how to manage their diseases, promoting exercise, discussing options for a healthy diet, or considering complementary therapies. Nurses have the added advantage of working with patients on a day-to-day basis and providing care for activities of daily living. This helps them to understand better the normal routines of certain patients and how they can incorporate wellness activities into daily living. Nurses are also connected to other members of multidisciplinary teams and often work with several groups who also promote total patient wellness. By connecting with others, nurses can provide additional resources to patients across several disciplines, which work toward promoting total patient care.

36

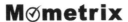

ADVANCED GENERALIST

Clinical nurse leaders act as **advanced generalists** insofar as they have advanced education in nursing, yet remain at the front line of care. Advanced generalists act as coordinators of patient-care plans, interacting with patients and their families to best serve their needs through clinical expertise. Clinical nurse leaders must be able to make clinical care decisions, use critical thinking skills to analyze risks and quality improvement, and use current nursing technologies to organize and provide patient care. Advanced generalists provide clinical education for both families and staff about various disease processes, cultural diversity needs, and performance improvement. Clinical nurse leaders communicate essential information among the various groups with whom they are involved, including staff, patients, families, physicians, and the interdisciplinary team.

CLINICAL NURSE LEADERS VS. NURSE PRACTITIONERS

While both **clinical nurse leaders and nurse practitioners** are required to have master's degrees in nursing, there are differences between the two types of nurses. The role of clinical nurse leaders is designed to improve the quality of patient outcomes, to act as liaisons for staff and physicians, to practice in the clinical setting, and to serve the nurses with whom they work. However, clinical nurse leaders are not designated as advanced practice registered nurses as nurse practitioners are. Nurse practitioners have been trained in a specific specialty, such as family practice, pediatrics, or psychiatric care. Nurse practitioners are able to prescribe medications for patient use, while clinical nurse leaders are not. In many areas, nurse practitioners may also work independently at their own facilities, while clinical nurse leaders must work under the authority of an organization or management system.

STANDARDS OF PRACTICE

The American Nurses Association has developed **standards of practice** that are consistent for all registered nurses. These standards are used to describe the values and priorities of nurses in their work, and they demonstrate the competencies of nurses who perform them correctly. Some examples of practice standards include performing patient assessments by considering health histories and physical condition, developing a nursing diagnosis based on the patient's condition, implementing interventions according to the patient's diagnosis, evaluating the effectiveness of nursing interventions, and determining outcomes that will best meet patients' needs. Additionally, for advanced practice nurses, they may act as nurse consultants to assist others in their work, or they may prescribe medications or therapies as part of treatments.

DETERMINING CONTINUED COMPETENCE

Clinical nurse leaders use various methods to **maintain professional competency**. Competency involves learning new measures and applying that knowledge to practice. Nurses may use continuing education to retain competency, which might be through classes, conferences, or other seminars to earn credit and to learn new methods of practice. Gaining professional certification in an area of expertise is another method of continuing competencies. Certification involves study, proof of professional practice, and testing to gain the associated credentials. Some positions also expect nurses to maintain portfolios of their work to demonstrate professional competencies through classes, presentations, or volunteer work.

NATIONAL REGISTRY OF CONTINUED COMPETENCE

Nursing competencies may vary between states, and while some organizations have developed standards for nursing competencies, there are few national standards that govern nursing practice throughout the entire United States. There are thousands of nurses working in various capacities throughout the country, and to attempt to establish the same competencies for all would be very difficult. Nurses work in a number of different clinical areas and specialties; what some nurses know and understand in one area may be vastly different from others. Also, there are nurses at all levels of competency because of experience: some nurses have graduated from nursing programs within the last 5 years, while others have decades of experience in practice. Finally, if a program could determine competency for all nurses across the nation, it would be very difficult to evaluate its effectiveness because of these factors.

LEVELS OF NURSING COMPETENCY

The level of nursing competency on a particular unit affects how patients receive care and the acuity level of patients that will affect care that is given. Nursing competency may vary between a nurse who has the skills and capabilities to perform the necessary work of the unit to one who is an expert clinician and who guides others in their work. **Competent nurses** are those who understand the care plan, can use clinical judgment to make decisions, are aware of patient rights, provide advocacy, maintain the safety of patients, and follow clinical guidelines. Alternatively, **expert nurses** may lead multidisciplinary approaches to patient care, change policies to reflect needs in certain patient populations, sense distinct changes in patients' conditions that require intervention, educate and mentor other staff, and perform or analyze research to improve patient-care standards.

PROFESSIONAL DEVELOPMENT

Professional development is something all nurses must consider as part of keeping up with their career. When planning for professional development goals, nurses should first identify those areas where they want to further their education or understanding of certain concepts. They may discover that there are some areas that need more work than others. It is important to then plan how they will work to attain these goals, such as taking continuing education courses, planning to attend seminars and presentations, or performing research. Once it has been decided what needs to be done to meet the goals, the activities can then be pursued. Afterward, nurses can evaluate how well the activities helped them in planning for professional development. Any courses, seminars, or certifications completed should be documented so that there is a record of their achievements.

CONTINUING EDUCATION

Continuing education is the practice of continued learning, after graduation from college or a nursing program. Nurses must perform continuing education as part of lifelong learning; additionally, many continuing education programs are designed to provide education as part of the credits needed to maintain licensure. Continuing education may be available through classes where nurses learn from an instructor. Classes may be offered through community college courses, seminars, conferences, or meetings. There may be tests following the presentation that determine how well the nurse understands the information. Continuing education may also be offered online or through self-study courses, which are similar to online courses, and may be offered through colleges, as webinars, through videos or slide show presentations, or as other forms of media. Again, nurses taking the courses often must take tests at the end of the session to determine competency.

GOAL ATTAINMENT

Developing professional goals is a pertinent aspect of the nursing profession. The process of setting and reaching goals prevents a nursing career from becoming stagnant and promotes lifelong learning within the field. When goal seeking, nurses should consider their future and attempt to set reasonable and measurable goals; they can then find out what arenas are available to help them to reach their goals, such as community education, seminars, conventions, or professional organizations. Nurses can then use these methods to work toward their goals, continuously

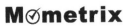

evaluating their progress and breaking the goals down into smaller steps, if necessary. Once they have reached their goals, they can evaluate the outcomes to determine the success of the process, and then commit to making new goals so they continue to move forward.

GIVING FEEDBACK WHILE TRAINING NURSES

When working with nurses who are in training, it is important for nurse leaders to provide **feedback** that is honest and direct yet sensitive. Effective feedback for nurses in training is constructive, rather than harsh. If negative information must be given, it should be delivered in a manner that offers a learning opportunity. Feedback should be specific, so that if changes are necessary, they are obvious. Nurse leaders should provide feedback in a timely manner, rather than waiting long periods to review the new nurse's work. If new nurses have issues in certain areas, clinical nurse leaders help them to develop a plan of action that addresses those issues. After implementing the plan of action, nurse leaders later evaluate the success of the plan, how well the nurses are responding, and whether the plan needs to be modified.

WRITING AN ARTICLE

When clinical nurse leaders write an article related to health or nursing activities, they often publish the article so that others can learn from their experience. The process of writing material for publication involves deciding on a topic that will be of interest to others. The information should be timely and relevant to nursing clinical practice. Nurse leaders can outline the information that they want to present and then write the data into journal or article form. Pictures and graphs that create visual representations of the data can be included. After writing the piece, the nurse leaders submit their manuscript to a journal or periodical for publication. If the piece is accepted, they may need to accept the terms offered by the publisher, which vary from company to company. When the articles are published, credit for their work is given, and clinical nurse leaders have the satisfaction of their work in print.

COLLABORATING WITH OTHERS TO DISSEMINATE INFORMATION

The CNL can **collaborate** with others to disseminate information and grow the profession. Opportunities include:

- **Team meetings**: The CNL can model collaboration by seeking input from other members of the team, showing respect for others, and sharing information, such as trends in medicine and evidence-based practice.
- **Board of directors/Administration**: The CNL can give formal presentations about the role of the CNL and advantages to the organization.
- **Community health care providers**: The CNL can meet with public health and other health care providers to discuss mutual needs and assist with problem-solving and health prevention efforts.
- **Professional organizations**: The CNL can take an active role in promotion of the profession by serving on committees, helping to organize events, and giving presentations.
- **Research opportunities**: The CNL can apply for grants when appropriate, carry out research, collect data, and report findings in conferences, team meetings, and/or publications.
- **Community groups**: The CNL can serve as a resource person for community groups, such as service clubs and school organizations.

Lateral Integration of Care Services

LATERAL INTEGRATION

Because health care is often fragmented, with many different professionals (nurses, occupational therapists, respiratory therapists, physical therapists, mental health counselors) providing care but with little contact or communication among them, increasing the risk of errors, the CNL serves a vital role in **lateral integration** (integrating different disciplines involved in clinical quality). In addition to fragmented care, patient stays in hospitals have shortened, requiring more services to be packed into a shorter duration of time. The role of the CNL as a lateral integrator includes:

- Coordinating patient activities and care.
- Meeting directly with the various professionals involved in patient care.
- Sharing information among the health care team.
- Overseeing the clinical care of the patient to ensure positive outcomes.
- Ensuring effective hands-off procedures.
- Intervening when necessary to ensure patient welfare.
- Reviewing all laboratory work and imaging studies to ensure important information is not overlooked.
- Ensuring patient/family receive necessary information and education.
- Assisting with development of the plan of care and discharge plan.

CLINICAL NURSE LEADERS AS LATERAL INTEGRATORS

Clinical nurse leaders have an important role as **lateral integrators** who work with nurses and staff who provide bedside care. While managers may be available to lead staff in decision-making, staffing needs, or financial issues, the primary role of clinical nurse leaders is in the clinical setting. Clinical nurse leaders serve as lateral integrators by acting as liaisons between disciplines to provide assistance to staff nurses and patients. Clinical nurse leaders facilitate discussions, collaborate with other disciplines, and serve as resources for staff to arrange appropriate services for patients on the units where they work. As lateral integrators, clinical nurse leaders work to reduce communication barriers between disciplines or between nurses and their patients and families. Clinical nurse leaders also take measures to facilitate organized and timely patient care among staff nurses. Clinical nurse leaders are unit based, in that they work in a specific area or microsystem, which is their clinical focus

PROMOTING THE SAFETY OF PATIENTS

Promoting the safety of patients is one role of clinical nurse leaders as lateral integrators, as the safety of patients requires the work of several disciplines and timely follow-up to ensure appropriate outcomes. Clinical nurse leaders may facilitate meetings between caregivers across all disciplines responsible for patient care, such as nursing, medicine, social services, or physical therapy. These meetings focus on such topics as safety practices, areas of concern, and policies that need to be remedied. Clinical nurse leaders also meet with staff from other areas, such as housekeeping, maintenance, or allied health support staff. Clinical nurse leaders consider policies that may need to be revised and work to make the appropriate changes by meeting with nursing managers or supervisors. Clinical nurse leaders also track incident reports to discern areas of weakness on the clinical units to determine what changes need to be made to prevent future errors.

CARE COORDINATION

Care coordination is the process of organizing patient care, which may involve various providers to provide adequate services. Within the clinical environment, care coordination may involve working with interdisciplinary teams to ensure that patients' needs are being met through several disciplines. Nurses who are care coordinators may need to contact several providers to communicate patients' needs; these nurses may meet with providers or arrange for them to meet patients. In addition, care coordinators may need to set up appointments for patients, may advocate for services, or may communicate with other providers if patients are unable to do so themselves.

POSITIVE OUTCOMES

Care coordination involves arranging services and coordinating patient care across more than one discipline. There are several **benefits** to both patients and nurses. Overall, care coordination increases communication among providers so that patients are more aware of the providers' roles in their care. This may reduce the frequency of unnecessary visits to providers, such as emergency room visits. It may foster greater involvement with patients in their own care, which reduces medical expenses from missed appointments or failure to use devices or therapies correctly. Patients may feel a greater sense of satisfaction that nurses are truly meeting their needs. Patients may also be more likely to have positive clinical outcomes when their care is managed through coordination, which reduces some of the responsibilities for nurses and may increase job satisfaction to know that patients' needs are being met.

PATIENT INVOLVEMENT

Nurses should always advise patients to become involved in making decisions for their own health and wellness. Nurses can recommend steps that will help patients to be engaged with health care providers and to become active members of the interdisciplinary team that is concerned with their health. Nurses can advise patients to research carefully their own health conditions, including treatments and medications, through valid sources. When patients have upcoming appointments, nurses can recommend that they come armed with questions about their care, ask about how tests are performed, when results are expected, and if they can receive written instructions. Patients should stay in contact with physicians or nurses to ensure that they are following treatment orders appropriately and that their questions regarding treatments are answered.

BARRIERS IN COORDINATING PATIENT CARE

Care coordination involves organizing the needed services for patients, which may be necessary through several disciplines. There are several **barriers** that may occur as nurses attempt to coordinate patient care. In some cases, no logical course of coordination exists, making it difficult for nurses to understand exactly what their role should be. This disorganization is not only a barrier for nurses but also does not benefit patients because services may be missing. Nurses might also have difficulty contacting providers or making arrangements to meet. In some cases, transitional meetings are necessary to cover essential information about patients. The providers may have difficulty finding a time that works for everyone's schedule. The care coordinator may not have enough information to know what resources to give patients or who to contact, which often develops over time and practice. Finally, patients may reject the work of care coordinators, choosing not to get involved with services or participate in decisions.

LACK OF APPROPRIATE CARE COORDINATION

Care coordination involves work with multidisciplinary teams to ensure that patients' needs are met in a comprehensive manner. Members of the team facilitate their segment of care until the team completes the patients' care coordination. Care coordination that does not involve adequate communication between team members or that does not exist at all can result in issues that could be avoided. Lack of communication may mean that some tests or treatments are repeated unnecessarily or not ordered at all. If patients do not receive adequate education about their diagnoses and treatment plans, they may be confused about to whom to talk. Patients may seek

41

follow-up treatment inappropriately or may be more likely to need follow-up care because they do not adequately follow treatment directions. All of these situations also lead to increased costs for patients and the health care system when patients' comprehensive care is not managed correctly.

Patient Assessment

COMPREHENSIVE PHYSICAL ASSESSMENT

A **comprehensive physical assessment** is carried out methodically, moving from one system to another to ensure that all body systems are reviewed. The examination begins with a patient and family history and then a general survey that includes assessment of psychosocial status, substance abuse, and domestic partner violence, and measurements (height, weight), vital signs as well as assessment of pain level and nutritional assessment. System-based physical examination utilizes inspection, palpation, percussion, and auscultation, While the order may vary somewhat, the usually order of examination is:

- Skin, nails, and hair.
- Head, face, and neck.
- Eyes, ears, nose, mouth, and throat.
- Breasts and regional lymph nodes.
- Thorax and lungs.
- Heart and neck vessels.
- Peripheral vascular/lymphatic system.
- Abdomen.
- Musculoskeletal system (may include functional assessment).
- Genitourinary system.
- Anus, rectum, and prostate.

PROBLEM-BASED FOCUSED ASSESSMENTS

Patients often present with a myriad of health problems, so a **problem-based focused assessment** that focuses on finding a solution to chief complaints and current health problems can be effective. The problem-based focused assessment requires a thorough history to create a problem list. This approach does not preclude a complete exam, which might identify problems that the patient has neglected, but the focus remains on the problem list generated. The list should be prioritized to ensure that the most critical issues (blood in the stool) are thoroughly assessed before less critical issues (occasional insomnia). Once a problem is identified, then differential diagnoses are determined. With patients, especially adults, there may be a combination of physical and psychosocial elements to a problem. For example, urinary problems may relate to dehydration, lack of mobility, poor hygiene, medications, or disease. Appropriate diagnostic tests, further assessments, and interventions are completed as needed to diagnose and resolve problems.

HOLISTIC ASSESSMENT PROCESS

Holistic nursing care focuses on patients and their relationship to health, their environment, and their self-care. When viewing patients as part of holistic nursing care, nurses consider the total person: their physical, psychological, cognitive, spiritual, and social systems, and how they are connected. Nurses also consider how these factors are meaningful to patients and their experiences and background. Nurses encourage self-care by recognizing that patients have a responsibility to care for themselves; nurses use the personal beliefs, values, and practices of patients to promote self-care measures and changes in practices that support health and wellness.

HOLISTIC PATIENT ASSESSMENT

A **holistic assessment** includes various aspects of patients' backgrounds beyond their physical symptoms and current state. The developmental assessment considers the stages of development and whether patients met developmental stages appropriately while growing. As adults, a developmental assessment may include developmental milestones that are appropriate for life stage, according to Erik Erikson. A cultural assessment considers patient's culture, practices, beliefs, and values. A spiritual assessment includes patients' beliefs about life, a higher power, illness, death, dietary practices, and their personal support system through a religious establishment or group.

IMPORTANCE OF VITAL SIGNS

Because **vital signs** describe current activity of the heart, lungs, and body temperature, measuring these is considered vital, hence the name. Most commonly, vital signs consist of heart rate, respiratory rate, blood pressure, and temperature; however, oxygen saturation is sometimes also included. Nurses should assess patients' vital signs upon admission; according to facility policy for the patient's condition, such as once a shift; before and during invasive procedures; when administering medications or treatments that may affect the vital signs, and any time nurses feel that patients may be showing changes in their condition. Nurses should remember that while there are so-called normal parameters for vital signs, actual results vary slightly among patients.

PICO

The **PICO** acronym is a method of assessing patient status, a very basic form of the nursing process that is easy to remember.

- "P" stands for **population**; nurses not only assess the disease process with which the patient presents but also the characteristics of the patient that may be similar to a population of patients, such as the patient's age, gender, culture, and social conditions.
- "I" stands for **intervention**, which includes those actions the nurse takes to provide care and treatment. "I" may also include an assessment of the patient's risk for complications, such as hospital-acquired illness.
- "C" stands for **comparison**, which compares the patient's current disease process with other potential factors, complications, or conditions.
- "O" stands for **outcome**, which provides goals for patient care that should be evaluated on a consistent basis to determine whether the interventions are effective.

BRADEN SCALE FOR PREDICTING PRESSURE SORE RISK

The **Braden Scale for Predicting Pressure Sore Risk** was developed to assist nurses and caregivers to predict patients' susceptibilities to developing pressure ulcers. The scale is a tool that nurses may use to assess for factors that increase patients' risks, such as sensory perception, mobility, nutrition, activity levels, skin moisture, and the amount of friction on the skin. Patients at risk may be assessed through the Braden Scale, which gives a score for each area. Based on the total score, nurses can then assess patients' risks of developing an ulcer. If patients are at high risk, nurses can use preventive measures to prevent the development of an ulcer.

CLINICAL MICROSYSTEM ASSESSMENT

A **clinical microsystem** is a small team of health care providers who work together to provide health care to a specific group of patients, such as heart transplant patients. The purpose of the clinical microsystem assessment is to determine if the microsystem is working to maximum efficiency and achieving desired outcomes and to help to improve the quality of care. While assessment tools may vary, common elements include:

- **Leadership**: Leaders support performance goals through positive culture, clear expectations, and empowerment.
- **Support**: Organization is supportive, recognizes contributions, and provides needed resources.
- **Staff**: Team members are valued and respected; workloads and schedules are reasonable and equitable.
- **Education/Training:** Education is ongoing and reflects the needs of the microsystem.
- **Collaboration**: The team is interdependent and works well together, showing respect for everyone's contributions.
- **Patient**: Patient needs are anticipated and met.
- **Community**: Staff meet community needs and exhibit cultural competency.
- **Performance improvement**: Continual performance improvement is integral to the team with adequate resources to carry out data collection and studies.
- **Information/Technology**: Patients and team members have easy access to information needed and the technology necessary for access.

Ethics

ALTRUISM

Altruism involves caring for others in a selfless manner by considering the needs of others without expecting a reward in return. Nursing care must consist of an altruistic attitude, as nurses must be sensitive to the needs of patients and provide care in a sympathetic and responsive manner. Nurses practice altruism by taking time to recognize their patients' needs and to respond to them in a timely manner. They go above and beyond the minimum standards of their job to provide education or caring methods that patients may not have otherwise received. Many patients state they felt their nurses cared about them when they took the time to talk with them, arrange for special services, or were simply friendly and approachable. Nurses practice all of these things without the expectation that they will get anything in return from the patient or the family.

UPHOLDING PATIENT AUTONOMY

Autonomy refers to patients' rights to make their own decisions regarding their health. Autonomy describes patients' rights to self-determination; they have the ability to make choices about what type of treatment they want or how they want to manage their health. Clinical nurse leaders uphold patients' autonomy in the clinical setting by avoiding paternalistic attitudes that imply patients have little understanding or choice in their health. They can support autonomy by including patients in interdisciplinary meetings, discussing treatment decisions with them, and gaining informed consent. Clinical nurse leaders may also need to discuss treatment options with patients' families if they are involved. A part of upholding autonomy is helping patients to overcome challenges to their care and to support the decisions that they make, even if they differ from those of the nurses.

BENEFICENCE AND NON-MALEFICENCE

Beneficence and non-maleficence are two practices that are involved in the ethical care of patients among nurses.

- **Beneficence** is the process of doing good things for the sole benefit of others. Practicing beneficence is a core component of nursing care and is part of most actions nurses do to provide for patients. By practicing beneficence, nurses promote patients' health and well-being, as well as reduce those instances that might cause them harm.
- **Non-maleficence** means not doing things that would be harmful to patients. Nurses must seek to do well in all of their work and avoid those situations that are not effective parts of patient care or that specifically hurt patients.

DEMONSTRATING RESPECT

Demonstrating **respect** involves providing care that truly considers the needs of patients, nurses' coworkers, and themselves. Respect involves showing consideration for others as well as appreciating differences in a way that promotes kindness and equality.

- Nurses who demonstrate **respect for their patients** consider each person as someone of value with a specific background, medical condition, and set of beliefs about which the nurse cares.
- Nurses who **respect their coworkers** understand that all people with whom she works have their own needs, schedules, and personal backgrounds that should be considered. This involves helping and supporting others so that all workers can get along, work together, and regard each other's needs.
- Nurses who **respect themselves** recognize that they are people of worth and that they must maintain their own health and well-being to provide appropriate care for others.

VERACITY

Veracity refers to telling the truth; in health care situations, nurses have an ethical obligation to tell patients the truth about their conditions. This should occur even if patients do not have good prognoses, because patients have a right to know. Patients expect truthfulness from health care staff as part of seeking care and receiving treatment. Nurses often want to protect their patients from difficult information or data that may cause psychological upset. Nurses must consider what to tell patients according to their rights as people and what is useless information that will only cause harm. Telling the truth and sticking with the principles of veracity increase patients' trust in nurses to be honest and forthcoming with information.

BIOETHICS

Bioethics refers to studying how ethical issues may arise within science and medicine. Examples of bioethical issues abound in health care, and nurses may be placed in difficult situations that require them to make moral decisions while still upholding what is best for their patients. Some examples of bioethical issues include keeping important information from patients about their health because telling them the truth may cause psychological harm, helping family members involved with patient care when they refuse treatment that could be helpful or life-saving, assisting with patients who cannot make their own decisions and who do not have a medical power of attorney, or working with patients who do not understand their conditions due to language, cultural, or health-literacy barriers.

ETHICAL CODES

Ethical codes are guides that are given to direct appropriate behavior and response when ethical dilemmas are encountered. Ethical codes define morals or beliefs that should be followed in questionable situations. Although ethical codes provide guidelines, there is not only one right answer for every situation, and these codes cannot answer every ethical problem by providing sets of rules. Alternatively, virtue ethics focuses on the moral behavior and character of the people involved with making ethical decisions. Nurses who have virtuous qualities are more likely to make moral decisions in the face of ethical dilemmas. If nurses do not possess virtue ethics, they may not make moral decisions in ethical situations, even if ethical codes are in place.

CODE OF ETHICS APPLIED TO ALL NURSES

A **code of ethics** is designed to apply to nurses at all levels of education and practice, regardless of the amount of time they spend providing patient care. Because nursing positions often involve a variety of practices, involving patients receiving direct care in hospitals and health organizations or those in the community, nurses at many different levels have the potential to impact the health and ethical decisions of their patients. Nurses who are in positions to make decisions, such as those who implement staffing procedures, those who work in quality or risk management, or those who work in fiscal departments, are still obligated by a code of ethics because their work indirectly affects patients. Advanced-practice nurses are often responsible for making decisions that affect patients and are also bound by a code of ethics. Nursing as a profession is created to serve many different populations of patients by following ethical codes of conduct, whether patient care is direct or indirect.

ENCOUNTERING ETHICAL ISSUES

Nurses have several responsibilities that are considered fundamental to their practice, including **promotion of health and alleviation of suffering**. These principles may create ethical dilemmas in practice if nurses encounter situations that clash with what they know to be part of their responsibilities and obligations. Promoting health is fundamental to nursing in that nurses are responsible for educating patients about their health and encouraging habits that promote wellness and prevent disease. However, some nurses may encounter ethical dilemmas while promoting health among their patients if they are supporting or encouraging practices that clash with the cultural or religious beliefs of certain groups. Alleviating suffering is another component of basic nursing responsibility, but in some situations, the attempt to provide comfort may result in an ethical dilemma, such as in the case of managing pain among terminally ill patients. Nurses must understand their own roles as caregivers to handle these situations when they occur.

CONFLICT OF INTEREST

A **conflict of interest** occurs when there is a disagreement or competition between two different interests. In many cases, people are faced with a conflict of interest when they need to make a decision and are being influenced by one position over the other. Nurses can avoid coming into conflicts of interest by remembering that patient care is their top priority, rather than serving the needs of others. They should be honest about any attempts at influence to notify those involved that they will not be manipulated. Nurses may avoid situations in which a potential conflict of interest could arise, such as by avoiding events where gifts to nurses might be given. If nurses encounter pressure from an entity that could result in a conflict of interest, they should report the matter to their managers or to the administration.

TRANSPARENCY

Nurses may encounter situations in which they must manage potential conflicts of interest. When this happens, there is risk of being influenced by certain companies or authorities to make decisions that result in a particular outcome. **Transparency** involves being open and honest about these potential conflicts to ensure that there is nothing occurring that would even be questionable. This transparency is important among different groups. For example, transparency must be extended to health care professionals by outside organizations to let nurses and staff know that they will not try to influence their decisions through persuasion or gifts. Transparency is also important for nurses to demonstrate by disclosing information that may be objectionable, such as financial ties with certain organizations, in which there could be misunderstandings about potential conflicts of interest.

END-OF-LIFE DECISION-MAKING

End-of-life decision-making is the process of making decisions that may or may not prolong patients' lives; it is a decision made by patients' caregivers, physicians, and families. End-of-life decision-making may involve whether or not to use treatments that may extend patients' lives or whether no further measures should be taken. There are times when patients have advance directives and have appointed guardians to make legal decisions for them in case they become incapacitated. In these cases, the health care providers must legally follow the instructions for end-of-life care. Nurses might also face patients' wishes regarding resuscitative efforts; in some cases, patients have signed do-not-resuscitate orders. Finally, nurses may encounter decisions regarding withdrawing life support for some patients who require ventilation or medications in order to stay alive.

PEACEFUL DEATH

Nurses can have an important impact on the **environment of dying** patients to make it as peaceful as possible. They may allow and encourage family members to stay with patients, including providing an extra bed in the room for family members. Nurses might allow patients' families to bring in meaningful items or to play soft soothing music. Keeping the environment quiet, limiting extraneous noise from the unit, and reducing interruptions can all promote a peaceful environment. Nurses should manage patients' pain and keep them comfortable. They should be aware of patients' wishes, particularly advance directives, so that they can perform care in accordance with the desires of patients. Finally, nurses should remain available to patients and their families to ensure that their needs are met for information and help.

BARRIERS TO A PEACEFUL DEATH

Because nurses are typically at the forefront of patient care, they may be one of the parties most involved with helping patients through the dying process. Although most nurses want to be able to provide a peaceful death for patients, there are several **barriers** that may occur. Often, nursing shortages do not allow nurses to focus on one patient because they may be assigned to several patients, even in a critical care unit. Communication issues are another reason why death and dying may be difficult, as nurses struggle to get a hold of physicians to explain what is happening or to help family members understand what is going on. Nurses may encounter unrealistic expectations about patients' deaths that may result in feelings of frustration and disappointment on the part of patients' and their families. Finally, a misunderstanding about patients' wishes or advance directives can impede a peaceful death when health care providers are forced to interpret patients' desires for how they wish to die.

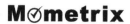

INTERDISCIPLINARY TEAM ETHICAL CONSIDERATIONS

Nurses are working with patients with increasingly complex diagnoses, requiring increased participation on interdisciplinary teams. When sharing information among team members, nurses need to consider several items that may breach ethical standards. All members of the team have their own duties and obligations, and all must stay within the confines of their scope of practice when making decisions. Team members should also act in a respectful manner toward each other, which is not only ethical, but fosters a productive work environment. Because there may be team members who have different levels of responsibility and professional status, such as physicians working with nurses, who may in turn work with medical assistants, all team members must bring their own strengths to the meeting to add to the cohesiveness of the group.

PROFESSIONAL PRACTICE BOUNDARIES

As part of upholding ethical practice and moral decision-making, nurses are expected to maintain certain **professional practice boundaries** to protect patients and support clinical practice. Examples include being authentic in relationships with other nurses, being authentic and accountable to patients and their families, and showing honesty in practice when working with other practitioners, such as physicians or those on interdisciplinary teams. Additionally, nurses should avoid inappropriate relationships with patients or their families; for example, they should not accept personal gifts from patients for providing care, they should maintain patient confidentiality and privacy, and they should not knowingly put patients into situations that might cause a breach of ethical standards.

HEALTH CARE FRAUD

Health care fraud is an illegal activity that occurs when individuals intentionally deceive the health care system for their own personal gain. Health care fraud could take several forms, including falsification of records, over- or undercharging for medical services, misrepresentation as a health care provider when one is not licensed or educated to practice, purposefully inaccurately billing companies for payment of services, forging signatures of health care providers, sending claims to insurance companies for incorrect services or services that were never provided, or assuming another person's identity for the purpose of receiving health care. If nurse leaders determine that someone is committing health care fraud, they have a duty to report the fraud to the proper authorities. Depending on the situation, this entails reporting the violation to the supervisor, to the medical board, to the hospital administration, to the associated insurance companies, or to the Federal Bureau of Investigation.

NEGLIGENCE

Within health care, **negligence** is defined as performing any act of omission or commission that a reasonable person would otherwise not do. Negligence in practice refers to the duties that nurses are expected to perform as part of their work, and they either do not do them or do them incorrectly. Negligence may often result in harm to patients. Some examples include giving the wrong dose of medication, mistaking patients' identities, or failing to protect patients in certain situations so that injuries result. Nurses can avoid being negligent by carefully checking all medications; performing the five rights before administering any medication; carefully delegating responsibilities, so that they do not entrust care to inappropriate personnel; thoroughly documenting their activities; correctly following the policies of the hospital; obtaining appropriate consent in mandated situations; taking measures to maintain the safety of patients; and taking clear orders from physicians.

ETHICS COMMITTEE

An **ethics committee** serves several roles in the organization with which it is affiliated, and education of patients and staff is one of them. The ethics committee provides education to staff and the community about ethical issues, particularly those that are current or more common than others. The committee also acts as a resource for others to provide information for when they are managing ethical conflicts. They may provide basic education for certain procedures, such as legal proceedings or maintaining privacy information. The ethics committee may provide educational offerings at their location or within the community to larger groups, or they may visit smaller settings, agencies, long-term care facilities, or clinics. Their educational goals are to provide comprehensive education to anyone who manages ethical issues, including bioethics, cultural practices, quality of life issues, spiritual aspects, or legal issues.

NURSE AS A MEMBER OF THE ETHICS COMMITTEE

An ethics committee may be available at a health care organization specifically for the purposes of advising and assisting with decisions that cause ethical dilemmas. An ethics committee may consist of several members of the interdisciplinary team, including physicians, social workers, nurses, clergy, or attorneys. Each of these professionals bring their expertise to the team to assist with decision-making that involves ethical dilemmas. Nurses bring a unique perspective to the ethics committee in that they are often at the forefront of patient care. They may be directly involved with patients or families with the ethical dilemma. They may be the people who initially bring the problem to the committee or may have the responsibility to educate patients and staff about the results of the committee's discussion. Through an ethics committee, nurses work with various team members to make appropriate decisions that are ethically sound and in the best interests of patients.

ETHICAL DECISIONS

Ethics committees are asked to consult on various decisions in which they must consider the issue itself, the effect on patients and families, and any legal ramifications that are involved. When discussing a case, the committee must review the associated medical records and talk about the situation with the caregivers and patients. When considering a decision in a case, an ethics committee must also take into account patients' health and prognosis, patients' cognitive capacities and abilities to make decisions, available treatments and alternatives, the financial implications of the decision, the quality of life for patients, and the amount of pain or suffering involved. Additionally, the committee must also consider factors such as patients' wishes, the presence of advance directives, and patients' abilities to make competent decisions with the full understanding of the situation.

Clinical Outcomes Management

Epidemiological Patterns

EPIDEMIOLOGY

Epidemiology is the study of disease within a population. The nurse epidemiologist may be focused on one specific type of disease or work on a broader scope within public health. Because disease spread and infection can affect so many different aspects of human life, nurses often partner with those in other disciplines to determine how certain diseases begin, how their rates of spread are affected, and how the results are analyzed. They often must work with others outside of health care, including statisticians to provide analysis of data, geographers to study disease distribution, biological scientists who determine how the disease affects the environment, and demographers who study how the disease affects the human population.

AGENTS

Agents are items that cause or contribute to disease conditions. When nurses study disease-causing mechanisms, they must consider how agents affect hosts to cause disease.

- **Biological agents** are those that may or may not be infectious; they are often organisms in the form of bacteria, viruses, or fungi that cause disease.
- **Psychological agents** are typically those that affect mental health that can contribute to disease, such as stress.
- **Physical agents** include those means that might occur environmentally, such accidents or natural disasters.
- **Nutritional agents** impact the body based on the patient's nutrient intake, such as a vitamin deficiency or toxicity.
- A **chemical agent** is often a substance that contributes to disease, such as industrial chemicals or pesticides.

SPREAD OF INFECTION

Nurses and clinicians now better understand how many diseases are spread, including infections in the clinical setting. Because of this knowledge, measures are implemented to control the spread of bacteria and viruses that may infect patients and cause disease. Within the clinical setting, infections such as wound infections, ventilator-associated infections, or septicemia may originally develop because of a triad of factors. The patient represents the host for the agent that is causing the infection. The agent enters the patient's body and spreads, resulting in disease. The agent of infection is often a certain type of bacteria, virus, fungus, or spore. The environment contributes to the spread of the infection, such as situations in which people do not wash their hands, surfaces are not appropriately sanitized, or nurses do not use sterile technique with invasive procedures.

ACTIVE IMMUNITY

Active immunity refers to resistance to certain types of disease. This resistance occurs through the environment or in some cases, it can be promoted through active measures. When it occurs naturally, active immunity may be the result of exposure to a specific disease against which patients then produce antibodies for future protection. This natural immunity is often uncontrolled, but after surviving an infection, patients may benefit from never succumbing to it again. Alternatively, nurses can also promote active immunity by immunizations, which provide a small amount of exposure to infection so that the body produces antibodies for future protection. Nurses can

50

promote vaccinations by recommending that patients receive their seasonal influenza shots, educating parents about the importance of childhood immunizations, or teaching patients about the schedule to receive vaccinations.

HEALTH TRAJECTORY

The term **health trajectory** refers to the course of an illness or condition of patients. Nurses often witness patients' health trajectories during their course of care in the clinical unit. Through documentation, nurses may be able to identify or predict certain patterns on health trajectories, which could change the nurses' course of action. For example, nurses may document patients' vital signs and note that over the past several hours, blood pressure has been slowly dropping. This may lead to close monitoring or other responses from nurses, depending on the patients' acuity. Review of documentation gives clues about patients' conditions that may lead to negative changes, which require nurses to change their practices. Because of changing health trajectories, nurses may need to change their interventions, notify physicians, or provide further education for patients.

CHRONIC ILLNESS AND ENVIRONMENT

The **environment** has a distinct effect on the brain, and responses to environmental stimuli may cause certain reactions within the body. Traumatic environmental impacts may result in the fight or flight response, which is the reaction of the sympathetic nervous system. The brain may perceive certain risks in the environment that will affect its response and, in turn, the response of the body. When these environmental factors have persisted over time, the brain repeats its responses to triggers. Ultimately, these responses could lead to chronic psychological illness as a result of changed patterns in the nervous system. For example, people exposed to traumatic events in their environment may develop a pattern of responses that appear exaggerated in everyday life but are actually very real to the people experiencing them. These responses then can lead to chronic and debilitating conditions, such as depression and anxiety.

Care Plan Development and Evaluation

CURRENT CARE PLAN

Nurses develop **patient-care plans** shortly after their first encounter with patients. The plan of care is developed based on the patients' assessment outcomes, histories, and reasons for seeking care. Nurses use this information to formulate appropriate nursing diagnoses and list interventions that are associated with the diagnoses. Ultimately, nurses develop goals or outcomes that patients should meet while under their care. The care plan must be evaluated frequently to determine if interventions are appropriate and if patients are responding and working toward the specified outcomes. If not, the plan of care may need to be revised to reflect the current status of patients. The care plan should be accessible to other members of the team who may also be caring for the same patients, so that all staff are up-to-date about the patients' diagnoses, needed interventions, and outcomes.

STANDARDIZED-CARE PLANS

Standardized-care plans can be used for more than one patient. These care plans may be beneficial in environments where patients are seen for similar conditions and whose nursing diagnoses, interventions, and outcomes are comparable. Standardized-care plans give nurses automatic access to what measures they need to take and what interventions are necessary. Using standardized-care plans also may save nurses time spent in developing a plan of care from the beginning. They give nurses ideas for what to expect with certain patients, supporting critical thinking skills and monitoring processes. Although standardized-care plans are beneficial in many ways, nurses must still consider patients as individuals and may need to change the care plan to fit their needs.

WRITING PATIENT GOALS FOR TREATMENT

Patient outcomes are an essential part of the nursing care process. When writing about nursing outcomes, nurses not only need to understand the needs of patients, but they should create goals that are individualized. The outcomes should be specific to patients' particular needs, and they should be measurable so that nurses can determine their effectiveness later when evaluating success. Nurses should use evidence-based practices to formulate their goals so that outcomes coincide with current standards. Goals should be realistic and attainable; setting unreasonable outcomes may set patients up for failure, and then outcomes must be revised. Finally, nurses must communicate with patients about what their outcomes are so that patients can actively participate in working toward their goals.

PATIENT OUTCOMES AND NURSING DIAGNOSIS

Outcome identification differs from the nursing diagnosis portion of the nursing care process. Outcomes guide nurses for what interventions they must use, serve as goals for providing patient care, and are used to evaluate the effectiveness of the nursing care plan. Alternatively, nursing diagnoses shape what the outcomes will be. They are used as guides for how nurses eventually evaluate their nursing care based on patients' conditions. Nursing diagnoses are often contrary to the outcomes; for example, a nursing diagnosis of "impaired skin integrity" should have an outcome of "maintaining intact patient skin."

LONG-TERM AND SHORT-TERM OUTCOMES

Outcomes for patients may be based on time, and the time it takes to achieve certain outcomes is dependent on the patient's condition, the nursing diagnosis, and the nurse's interventions for patient care.

- **Long-term outcomes** may involve more than a week of work for the patient. Long-term outcomes may also be used to evaluate the overall nursing care through the patient's length of stay or as part of the dismissal evaluation.
- **Short-term outcomes** are typically less than a week in length and may only last a few days or even a few hours, depending on the patient's condition.

TYPES OF OUTCOME CATEGORIES

Although outcomes are designed to determine intervention effectiveness for patients, outcomes may be further divided into patient-focused outcomes and provider-focused outcomes, based on the processes involved to reach the goals.

- **Patient-focused outcomes** are those associated with the patient's physical processes, such as how the body responds to certain types of treatments, the physiological progression of disease within the body, changes in body processes as responses to interventions, or changes in emotional status as a result of cognitive-behavioral therapy.
- **Provider-focused outcomes** are related to those activities that nurses perform to help patients reach their goals. Provider-focused outcomes might be effective patient care, nursing knowledge of the clinical situation, nursing competence in skills, and recognition of cultural variances.

MEDICAL DIAGNOSES AND NURSING DIAGNOSES

Patients who are receiving care and treatment often have both medical diagnoses and nursing diagnoses applied to their care.

- **Medical diagnoses** are provided by physicians and are based on patients' symptoms, history, and diagnostic tests. Medical diagnoses focus on treatments and control or elimination of the condition.
- Alternatively, **nursing diagnoses** are provided by nurses and are based on nursing assessments as well as potential outcomes surrounding the conditions of patients. Nursing diagnoses focus on patients, rather than on their conditions, and serve as holistic measures to ensure the patients' needs are met while they receive treatment. The nursing diagnoses also guide nurses for interventions that address the patients' situations, ultimately leading to outcomes designed as part of the nursing process.

KNOWLEDGE DEFICIT

Knowledge deficit is a nursing diagnosis commonly seen in patients in many different care units. Nurses who care for patients with a diagnosis of knowledge deficit should implement interventions that provide education about the patient-care plan, the diagnoses and treatments, and continuing evaluations. Some outcomes associated with knowledge deficit include patients finally understanding the process of treatment and their own role in treatment measures, plans by patients for knowing who to ask if they have questions regarding their medications, understanding how to respond to changes in their conditions, and the reasons for taking certain types of medicine or performing certain treatments. The outcomes should be individualized for patients and specifically measurable for their particular needs.

SELF-CARE DEFICIT

A nursing diagnosis of **self-care deficit** reflects the inability of patients to care for themselves. Nurses need to assess patients' needs before beginning interventions. Nurses may need to consider whether patients use mobility aids for movement or how much they are able to do on their own. Nurses can then assist patients with tasks, allowing them to do as much activity as possible. Nurses may provide patients with assistive devices that enable them to perform tasks more easily. Nurses may provide assistance with hygiene, providing as much privacy as possible. If patients are unable to move around in bed, nurses must ensure that the objects patients need are within reach, such as the call light or the phone. Finally, nurses provide ongoing education to keep patients aware of their goals for activity and help them understand their role in pursuing optimal outcomes.

NURSING-SENSITIVE INDICATORS

Nursing-sensitive indicators are those patient care measures that affect the nursing process. Nursing-sensitive indicators are typically grouped into three different tools.

- **Structure indicators** describe the components of the nursing staff: their education and expertise, staffing ratios, or current certifications.
- The **process indicators** measure certain types of care that nurses may give, such as performing assessments, developing nursing diagnoses, and providing interventions.
- The **outcome indicators** help to determine the quality of patient care provided based on patient outcomes. These indicators may include such outcomes as infection rates, wound development, or patient falls, which reflect the scope of nursing care.

GOAL-ORIENTED PATIENT CARE OUTCOMES

Goal-oriented patient care outcomes focus on patients' well-being across several measures, including physical, emotional, and social health, as well as improving quality of life. The goal-oriented design focuses on patients as individuals, providing a holistic approach. The goal-oriented approach considers patients' particular situations to work on their outcomes, rather than viewing them as a group of people with the same condition. Patients are able to take part in deciding their own goals, thus providing more meaning to their care. This can make decisions about health a greater priority for patients. Because outcomes should be achievable and measurable, the goal-oriented approach allows nurses to evaluate fully their interventions to determine whether they are effective toward meeting patient outcomes.

EVALUATION PROCESS

During the **evaluation** stage of the care-plan process, nurses review the information in the patient's plan of care to determine whether interventions, goals, and nursing diagnoses are appropriate and are being met. If the information no longer applies to patients or the data are not specific, nurses can refine the care plan in the evaluation process. Some types of questions nurses may ask themselves during this process include:

- Are the included interventions appropriate for this nursing diagnosis?
- Are the interventions helping patients meet their goals?
- Are patient outcomes specific enough to their particular situation?
- Are patient outcomes realistic and attainable?
- Are there any interventions or nursing diagnoses that should be changed or added?

Coordinating Interventions

NURSING INTERVENTIONS

Nursing interventions are based on nursing diagnoses. Nursing interventions may be classified into different measures, depending on how they are performed and their effects on the patient. Monitoring activities involve checking on the patient to assess for changes in status, evaluating results of physical interventions, and analyzing the patient's health status over time. Instructing interventions include educating patients about their health or nursing practices and providing teaching to patients or families about important information surrounding the current care period. Referring interventions involve communicating with other providers and giving referrals as needed to other disciplines.

HOMEOSTASIS

Homeostasis describes certain processes that are in a state of balance within the body. Homeostasis, for example, can be assessed in body fluids, tissues, or cells. It is essential for nurses to understand appropriate electrolyte levels in the body to be able to recognize changes in patients that may indicate deterioration because of a lack of homeostasis. Nurses must help patients to maintain fluid intake, output, and overall fluid volume, which can affect electrolyte levels if not managed properly. Nurses record patients' intake and output to determine fluid status. They also must monitor electrolyte levels in laboratory results that can indicate too little or excessive electrolyte levels in the bloodstream, which could be dangerous for the patient. If electrolyte imbalances are detected, nurses report this information to the provider for further orders.

HOLISTIC NURSING CARE

Holistic nursing care focuses on the patient as a **whole person**, rather than simply treating symptoms or illnesses. Holistic nursing uses nursing knowledge to care for patients' physical, emotional, social, and spiritual well-being and to promote wellness. It is centered on the personal health of patients as opposed to various treatments or cures. Patients may choose to use both biomedical therapies used in Western medicine as well as alternative or complementary therapies. Nurses who provide holistic care create an environment of healing, support and empower patients regarding their own health, educate patients about their options for health and wellness, and help patients and their families to find meaning in the experience.

PHILOSOPHY OF HOLISTIC NURSING CARE

Holistic nursing considers the integration of health and wellness with each patient's experience. Holistic nursing recognizes several philosophies that are integral to its approach. It considers the spiritual background of each person and integrates this into care; it promotes self-care measures among patients by recognizing their responsibility to support their own health, and it values the cultural backgrounds of individuals by recognizing certain essential practices or beliefs. Holistic nursing also focuses on disease prevention and promotion of health; it recognizes the value of nursing care as part of the patient healing process; it may promote alternative or complementary therapies into nursing and medical care measures; and it considers the role of the environment on patients' abilities to care for themselves.

DEVELOPING HOLISTIC CARE PLANS

Developing a **care plan** is an essential nursing practice; when nurses are involved with holistic care, the care plan encompasses their patients' total system for mind and body wellness. Nurses at first consider patients' current conditions, their prescribed treatments, and the potential alternatives to traditional treatments when developing a plan of care. They assess their patients' physical, mental, and emotional health as well as their spiritual well-being when developing the nursing diagnoses based on their background. When formulating outcomes, nurses must consider all forms of treatment or therapies that patients would like to use for their care. Nurses implement interventions that support holistic care and then partner with patients for their care. Finally, nurses evaluate the effectiveness of these therapies and determine what areas need change and what fields have been successful.

EDUCATION ABOUT HOLISTIC CARE PRACTICES

Education is an essential component of nursing care, and when providing **education about holistic practices**, nurses must consider their own needs as well as those of their patients. Nurses who are inexperienced in holistic care practices may need to educate themselves about the topic before expecting to provide adequate care. They may attend classes, engage in learning online, or meet with others who practice holistically to learn more about the ideas, practices, and beliefs surrounding holistic care. Once nurses have a level of education and understanding about holistic care practices, they can then implement this segment of care into their health care teaching. This involves determining patients' views and beliefs about holistic care and then educating them about resources and practices that come with promotion of health and wellness in the holistic sense.

HOSPICE CARE AND PALLIATIVE CARE

Hospice and palliative care are options for people who have a life-threatening illness to make their final months and days as comfortable as possible. Although hospice and palliative care are often considered interchangeable, they are not the same. Hospice refers to care given to a person who has 6 months or less left to live. Hospice care may be provided within inpatient settings in hospitals, but it is more often given in patients' homes. Palliative care is provided for patients who are uncomfortable because of disease or its treatment. Palliative care provides comfort measures to patients by controlling pain or reducing stress associated with illness. Although many nurses provide comfort measures to patients in hospice, patients do not need to have a terminal illness to receive palliative care. Patients who receive treatments for their conditions may also benefit from palliative care nursing.

FAMILY CARE PLAN

In some contexts, nurses work with entire **families** to develop care plans that will best serve their needs. During the intervention stage of the nursing process, nurses working with families must help them to understand what issues require nursing care. For example, nurses may need to help families understand the importance of avoiding lead exposure to maintain safety within the home. Nurses must also direct the family toward the activities they can do themselves to support their health. In the lead example, nurses could guide the family toward determining the sources of lead around their home or having the home tested for unsafe levels. Nurses then support the families to work toward healthy living by assisting them with making appointments or helping them find opportunities for healthy activities.

INVOLVING THE FAMILY

Most patients have at least one family member who is involved with their care. For this reason, family members should be engaged in patient care, as appropriate, because these are the people who may be providing more care and follow-up after patients are discharged. Involving families has several **benefits**, including a better understanding of patients' backgrounds in that the families often can give information about patients when they are unable to do so themselves. Family members are often a source of comfort to patients and may provide extra care during times of stress or anxiety, which supports nurses' roles. Family members may assist with some activities of daily living for patients, such as helping them dress or eat. Families are also able to provide a connection with the environment outside the health care setting, by maintaining care of patients' homes and staying connected with others, which can be a source of comfort and security.

COMPLEMENTARY OR ALTERNATIVE THERAPIES

Patients may use various types of **complementary or alternative therapies** based on their personal preference, educational background, or culture. Nurses should be aware of and know how to work with to certain alternative therapies.

- **Natural products** include herbal remedies, vitamins, supplements, and dietary therapies. Patients should always disclose what natural products they are using in case these products interfere with traditional medications or therapies.
- **Movement** is used to promote health and mental or spiritual well-being. Examples of movement therapies include tai chi, the Feldenkrais Method, or Pilates.
- **Energy therapies** focus on energy fields surrounding the body as they affect health and wellness. Examples include magnets, Reiki, or acupressure.

NURSES' RESPONSIBILITIES IN COMPLIMENTARY THERAPIES

Some patients may wish to use complementary therapies as adjuncts to standard medical treatments, and nurses may assist these patients by providing therapy or helping patients to receive certain services. Before providing complementary therapy, nurses must consider what they know about these therapies and if they are competent enough to provide it. They should understand the process of providing the therapy, the expected outcome, and the risks and benefits involved. Nurses should also assess if patients are aware of any risks or benefits associated with these therapies. Nurses must assess patients' goals for the therapy. Before providing a complimentary therapy, nurses must also determine whether complimentary therapies are within their scope of practice, according to the rules of the hospital or clinic in which they work.

PERSONAL OR PSYCHOLOGICAL BENEFITS

Complementary therapies are increasing in popularity for patients who wish to use resources beyond traditional medicine. Complementary and alternative therapies may provide a number of **benefits** for patients, including personal benefits or those that improve psychological well-being.

- Some complementary therapies have **fewer side effects** than traditional medicine and can be used in place of traditional medicine.
- Complementary therapies may also **reduce feelings of anxiety** and may **promote self-care** among patients; patients may like the feeling of knowing they are doing everything they can to support their health by going "above and beyond" with therapies that complement traditional medicine.

RAPID RESPONSE TEAM

A **rapid response team** is a group of care providers, often from several disciplines, who respond to calls for patient assessments in potentially changing situations. The rapid response team is typically deployed before patients reach an emergency situation that would require calling a code for cardiopulmonary resuscitation. The team typically consists of nurses, respiratory therapists, pharmacists, physicians, or nurse practitioners, who can assess patients, monitor their conditions, order treatment measures, and prevent further deterioration. In many hospitals, nurses, patients, physicians, or even family members may activate the rapid response team. The team is deployed in any situation where the status of patients must be assessed for deterioration into a potentially critical situation.

CARE MANAGEMENT

Care management seeks to increase patients' abilities for self-care and focuses on getting patients the resources they need for their health. Care management integrates **community resources** to provide education to patients about their health and to find providers who will provide therapy or treatments. Care management also involves coordinating among providers to maintain appropriate lines of communication for patient care. It may mean advocating for the patient's needs, improving access to services, or encouraging follow-up care. Some patients have limited health-literacy skills and are unsure where to seek care, so they find care inappropriately, such as through emergency department visits. Care management may also help these patients to identify a medical home where they can find services when they are needed.

Pharmacology

MEDICATION ADMINISTRATION

The **five rights of medication administration** are implemented to uphold safety and to avoid potentially lethal mistakes that affect both patients and nurses. The five rights of medication administration have been devised for use in any situation in which nurses administer a medication and should be employed before, during, and after administration.

1. First, nurses ensure that they have the **right patient**; they check the patients' charts, room numbers, armbands, and ask patients to identify themselves.
2. Nurses then check that they have the **right medication** by reading the label and comparing it with the chart or the prescription.

57

3. They then check the for the **right dose** of the medication by reading the label and the order when preparing the drug.
4. Next, nurses confirm the **right time** for the medication by finding out when it was given last and its current schedule for use.
5. Finally, nurses determine the **right route** or how the medication is to be delivered.

PATIENT-CENTERED APPROACH

Medication administration must be adapted to consider patients through the process of prescribing, administering, and monitoring. Medication that is prescribed by a physician should not be prescribed without considering the patients' specific needs for that medicine: why they need to take it, what their dose should be, or what the goal of taking it is for them. If possible, the medication process should be simplified and as easy to remember as possible, especially for those patients who are taking multiple medications daily. Instructions should be clear and concise, avoiding a lot of jargon that could be misinterpreted. If necessary, an interdisciplinary approach may work to streamline the medicating process and to consider outcomes of use. The interdisciplinary team can prevent excessive prescribing of certain medications when there is good communication among providers.

ADVERSE REACTIONS TO MEDICATIONS

Adverse reactions are situations in which patients have negative or harmful responses to medication. Adverse reactions may cause minor illness or may cause significant reactions that could lead to major illness or even death. Some examples of adverse reactions to medications include allergic responses, such as hives, rashes, or wheezing; reactions related to the amount of the medication taken, such as when patients develop excessive symptoms of the drug's intended effect; iatrogenic responses, in which symptoms occur that are similar to illness, such as diarrhea; or toxicities, in which blood levels are excessively high and result in renal or liver impairment. Additionally, some patients may suffer from other symptoms that are a result of adverse drug reactions, including light sensitivity, kidney problems, or birth defects.

MEDICATION EDUCATION

Nurses often work with patients who take a number of medications, all of which could have potential adverse interactions, causing a number of different side effects. It is important that patients are **well-educated** about their medications to avoid adverse outcomes as a result of miscommunication. Nurses should provide education about taking medications exactly as ordered, being sure that patients understand dosages, side effects, and therapeutic outcomes. Nurses should also encourage patients to ask questions if they do not understand information about their medication, know where to get their prescriptions filled, and notify health care providers of all medications that they might be taking. Nurses should let patients know how long to take certain medications and what the effects might be if they suddenly stop taking them.

MEDICATION SAFETY

Medications may be widely prescribed and used in a variety of settings, leading to potentially dangerous outcomes when they are not managed or monitored correctly. Increasing medication safety involves monitoring the type, dose, frequency, and response of medications provided to patients and documenting these facts. If new providers begin to prescribe treatment, they should be informed of what medications patients are currently taking to avoid over-prescribing. If patients are discharged to home or another setting, they should be given clear information about what medications they are to continue taking after they leave the health care environment to avoid confusion and taking medicine inappropriately. Finally, if technology is available in the health care environment, such as through barcode medication administration, it should be used to promote safety among patients and to avoid errors.

CONTROLLED SUBSTANCES

Controlled substances are classified into categories, or schedules. The schedule in which a controlled substance is classified depends on the risk of a person becoming dependent, how effective it is as a medication, and whether it has the potential to be abused. The categories are ranked from level 1 to level 5.

- **Schedule 1** controlled substances have the highest likelihood of contributing to addiction or abuse; examples include LSD or heroin.
- **Schedule 2** drugs carry a risk of abuse as well as physical or psychological dependence; examples include many opioids.
- **Schedule 3** drugs may carry a risk abuse but are less of a risk than schedule 2 substances; examples include stimulants.
- **Schedule 4** substances have less risk of abuse but may cause psychological dependence; examples include benzodiazepines.
- **Schedule 5** medications are the least likely to cause abuse or dependence; an example of these drugs is an opioid mixed with another medication, such as cough medication.

ANTICIPATING COMPLICATIONS

Measures that can be used to **anticipate complications** include:

- **Vital signs**: Often the first indication of complications is a change in the vital signs and/or temperature, and the pattern of change may give a clue to possible problems. For example, increased temperature may indicate infection while increase BP and decreased pulse may indicate increased intracranial pressure.
- **Knowledge of disease progression**: Because most diseases follow a usual progression, awareness of the changes that may occur over time can help to take steps to prevent the changes, to prepare the patient for the changes, and to identify them early and minimize complications.
- **Knowledge of medication adverse reactions**: While medications may have myriad possible complications, an awareness of the most common adverse effects (nausea, vomiting, diarrhea, rash) can help to identify and treat them quickly. Specific adverse reactions common to particular medications, such as neutropenia with chemotherapy, should be routinely assessed.

Safe Transition

TRANSITION

Transition is defined as moving from one state to another. In the case of patient care, transition may involve the move from being a hospitalized patient to being discharged to home or to another facility. Patients being discharged may accept this transition with relief and satisfaction or with apprehension and fear. Nurses must help patients through this transition to get them to a point of acceptance. Nurses can do this by analyzing patients' behaviors to look for signs of anxiety, fear, anger, or relief. Nurses may need to provide education about patients' situations and why it is appropriate for them to move to the next phase. If necessary, nurses may also need to provide referrals for ongoing care through such measures as counseling or social services if patients are experiencing significant difficulties making the transition.

TRANSITION SPECIALISTS

Nurses working as **transition specialists** help patients to make decisions about their health and to feel empowered as they move from the health care environment to home. Because patients will not have as many health services at home as they have had in the health care environment, they need to understand how to care for themselves, make decisions regarding their health care, and continue with their treatment regimens. Transition specialists may meet with patients before discharge to discuss issues, concerns, and treatment plans. Transition specialists then provide resources for patients that can be used after they are discharged. Transition specialists may need to meet with an interdisciplinary team to ensure that the various aspects of patient care are covered before patients go home. Through education and coaching, transition specialists prepare patients for discharge and then follow up to determine how well they have transitioned to home.

HEALTH CARE TO HOME TRANSITION

The transition period for patients must be a time of adequate communication and use of resources to ensure that patients have the information they need to move from their current care center to home. However, there are many challenges associated with making transitions; for example, patients may face difficulties with prescribed medications that were readily available in the hospital but now must be purchased from pharmacies. This may lead to financial difficulties or gaps in medication regimens. Lack of communication may cause a failure to provide adequate notification among providers when patients are transferred or discharged. With poor communication, patients' needs for follow-up may not be met, and there may be areas that fall through the cracks.

INTEGRATING COMMUNITY RESOURCES

Patients often have many needs that are not met with medications and treatment when the patient is cared for in the community, so the first step of integrating **community resources** into care management is to thoroughly assess a patient's other needs through interview, observation, and review of patient's history, support systems, and socioeconomic status:

- **Food**: Food banks and faith-based organizations may provide food to those who cannot afford it.
- **Meal preparation**: Meals-on-wheels programs may help to provide nutritious meals for those who cannot cook.
- **Support system**: Faith-based programs and community volunteer programs (such as Friendly Visitors) may provide visitors and some personal assistance, such as transportation.
- **Financial need**: Social workers can assess the patient's eligibility for financial assistance or low-cost housing.
- **Housing**: Homeless shelters may provide shelter, low-cost housing (including Section 8) agencies may a provide affordable alternatives.
- **Transportation**: Public transportation systems provide various options for those who are disabled, often at reduced cost and may include door-to-door service.

SOCIAL NETWORKS AND DECISION SUPPORT MECHANISMS

Social networks have gained increasing importance in care management. Social media may be used to share information, such as news about an outbreak or new healthcare program, to compare different programs and gather information (such as assessing the different services available in the community), to train staff members, and to communicate. For example, text messages or tweets may be utilized to send reminders about appointments or programs. Websites or Facebook pages may provide information about an organization and opportunities for patients to comment. Patient internet portals allow patients access to their records.

Decision support mechanisms, such as software applications and clinical guidelines, help to ensure patient safety and quality patient care. Software applications, the most common type of support mechanism, help to review data and suggest diagnosis and/or treatment options. Decision support applications may be integrated with the electronic health record, issuing alarms (for problems) and notifications (such as lab results), helping to identify errors in dosage or treatment and to avoid duplications of tests and/or services.

Factors Influencing Health

PREDICTIVE HEALTH

Predictive health considers the potential effects of physical and emotional factors and how they will ultimately impact future health. Predictive health looks at healthy behaviors, genetic backgrounds, biomarkers, and social factors to determine how they will affect a person's health throughout the lifespan. By examining these factors, health care providers can then change their interventions to support healthy activities that may reduce the instances of negative outcomes and promote positive change. For example, a patient with a family history of diabetes who is overweight is at higher risk of developing diabetes. Predictive health considers this and other factors to make changes that might include additional education about the risks of diabetes, health and nutrition services, or weight-loss techniques to reduce the patient's risk of developing the disease.

DETERMINANTS OF HEALTH

Determinants of health affect a person's health from infancy through advanced age; they encompass various factors, including self-care, social circumstances, and physical environment. Some determinants of health include a patient's educational background, job, working environment, income, social standing, level of support from family and friends, housing conditions, neighborhood, and available modes of transportation. Additionally, a patient's health and wellness practices are determinants of health, as are a history of physical development, coping skills, gender, and cultural practices.

RESPONSE TO ILLNESS AND CARE INFLUENCES

Factors that influence response to illness and care include:

- **Ethnicity**: Patients and family's reactions to treatment and prevention may be influenced by their ethnicity and cultural, religious/spiritual beliefs. Different ethnic groups view the family and individual autonomy differently, so decisions about treatment may be made by other than the patient, such as by the eldest male in the family. Attitudes toward the causes of illness and appropriate interventions vary widely. For example, if a patient believes illness is caused by evil spirits, the patient is likely to have little faith in Western medical treatment.
- **Socioeconomics**: The society the patient operates within has established norms for behavior and often applies value and judgment to diseases, treatment, and preventive methods that influence the patient's attitudes. Social pressure to conform may influence the patient's behavior. Economic status may affect access to care.
- **Support systems**: Support of the friends and family, emotional and financial, is often critical to a patient's response to illness and treatment. Some may have a broad base of support that they can rely on while others may have none.

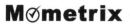

LOW HEALTH-LITERACY SKILLS

Low health-literacy skills indicate that patients have a limited understanding about medical information to make the best decisions for their health. It may not be obvious that patients have low health-literacy skills, so nurses should provide information in a way that is easy to understand without evoking shame in their patients. Nurses should avoid using medical jargon and instead speak clearly in plain language and short sentences. If available, pictures with basic information may be used to supplement the teaching. Nurses may need to assist patients with filling out forms or giving information regarding insurance and payments. When scheduling appointments, nurses should give patients the basic information that they need to know without adding a lot of other explanatory information. Complicated procedures should be explained using simple language. Nurses should use an interpreter if language is a barrier to ensure that information is communicated clearly.

RAPID ESTIMATE OF ADULT LITERACY IN MEDICINE TEST

The **Rapid Estimate of Adult Literacy in Medicine (REALM) test** is a test of adult literacy skills that can be administered quickly in certain situations to ascertain a person's knowledge of medical terms. The REALM test consists of 66 words that the person reads aloud while a test administrator scores the results. Scoring is based on the patients' abilities to pronounce words correctly as they move down the list. The list starts with words that have only one syllable and are easy to pronounce and progresses to complex, multisyllable words that are more difficult. Patients are scored based on the number of words that they correctly pronounce; scoring ranges from approximately third grade level to ninth grade level. The test can be administered in under 2 minutes.

MODIFYING EDUCATION BASED ON HEALTH LITERACY

Nurses frequently encounter patients with low health-literacy skills in their working environments, and it is important to understand the signs and know how to **provide education in a modified manner**. Because teaching and education are core components of the nursing profession, understanding health-literacy levels should be one of the main objects nurses can identify when beginning a teaching program with patients. However, many nursing programs do not include health-literacy topics or teach nurses how to identify those patients or families who appear to have low health-literacy skills. Clinical nurse leaders can implement this training topic when teaching new staff, whether they are recent nursing graduates or seasoned nurses who are new to the unit. They can determine the nurse's understanding of how to identify health-literacy skills among patients and provide education accordingly.

CULTURAL AND LANGUAGE BARRIERS

Nurses work with increasingly diverse populations with many different cultural beliefs and languages. Besides taking steps to adhere to patients' cultural values and provide language interpreters when necessary, nurses must also consider health literacy. Health literacy is the understanding patients have to be able to make informed decisions about their health and treatment. When cultural or linguistic barriers exist, health literacy disparities may also exist. Patients who do not understand the language of their health care provider may not fully understand medical terms needed to make decisions for their treatment. Patients who do not have the same cultural values as the health care provider may not have enough information to make their own health decisions. When addressing cultural and language barriers in patient populations, nurses need to address health literacy to ensure that they are not only reaching patients through their cultural background, but that they understand their health information as well.

PHARMACOGENOMICS

Pharmacogenomics looks at the genetic makeup of patients to determine which types of medication will work best with their genetic background. Pharmacogenomics can guide clinicians about how best to prescribe certain medications for patients' conditions. Through continuous research into the human genome project, pharmacogenomics may also give scientists the option of developing new drugs for some conditions and illnesses. This practice reduces instances of prescribing the same medications for all people with similar conditions and instead considers their genetic backgrounds to determine which medications are truly necessary. Some drugs are more or less effective in certain people, based on their genetic makeup.

BIOMARKERS

The term **biomarkers** is used to refer to biological markers that cause changes in the body, which guide clinicians in making decisions about care and treatment. Biomarkers can indicate changes in the tissues, at the cellular level, or in the bloodstream. These changes may direct clinicians to understand a patient's disease process, the potential for disease development, or the response of the patient to certain therapies or treatments. Biomarkers exist in various forms, including blood pressure, weight, or temperature. Biomarkers may also occur at the molecular level, indicating the potential for disease progression and assisting clinicians with early detection, such as biomarkers for breast or prostate cancer, or genetic testing for conditions such as cystic fibrosis.

CONCEPTS AFFECTING HEALTH BEHAVIORS

Several factors affect health behaviors and promote a healthy lifestyle among patients.

- **Attitude** is how the person views the situation; it could be positive or negative. In general, a positive attitude is more likely to promote change toward healthy behaviors.
- **Motivation** is the inner drive a person has for doing something. The person making lifestyle changes must have enough motivation to make changes toward meeting goals.
- **Self-monitoring** involves the person assessing changes and factors that affect health; it is a continuous process of evaluation to determine what actions are effective and what needs to be modified.

BELIEF SYSTEMS

Some patients, despite seeking treatment for their medical conditions, may not follow through with the necessary management of their illnesses. This is due to a variety of factors, including physiological, social, or emotional issues, but the belief patterns of patients may affect compliance with medical care. Many patients do not believe that their particular illness or condition will cause as many side effects or difficulties as they are told. This may be true in illnesses with few symptoms, such as hypertension. Other patients lack trust in the health care system or do not believe what physicians or nurses have told them about their conditions. Finally, some patients believe that their health is in the hands of a greater power and attempting to seek treatment may alter the will of this power.

DIVERSE BACKGROUNDS

Nurses working with various cultural groups may encounter patients with specific beliefs related to health care practices that are different from their own.

- **Magico-religious beliefs** are those that are centered on spiritual, religious, or magic forces that impact health and wellness. This belief system might consider the powers of other beings that affect health, whether because of punishment or through a testing process.

- With **deterministic beliefs**, patients believe that outside forces predetermine illness or injury, and there is no use in trying to fight it. Patients with this belief system might say, for example, "My illness is the will of God, and I won't try to prevent it."
- **Biomedical beliefs** are those that follow the idea that illness is due to system breakdown in the body, such as through genetic malformations or germ theory. Biomedical beliefs are consistent with those of most health care providers in the United States, which provide medical treatment for biological illnesses.

Health Promotion and Disease Prevention

COPING SKILLS

Nurses are at the forefront of patient care and often see varied responses to illnesses and diagnoses. Some patients do not possess adequate **coping skills** to handle their diagnoses, but nurses may be able to promote certain skills with some people to help them adjust. Nurses can encourage patients to get adequate rest and take good care of themselves by taking time to relax, exercise, eat right, or do enjoyable activities. They can counsel patients to talk about their condition further with a friend, family member, or member of the clergy; if available, they can offer to find groups of people struggling with the same condition. Nurses can encourage patients to express their feelings through journaling, self-reflection, and verbalization. Other coping skills include meditation, prayer, volunteering, keeping up with hobbies, and exercise.

HEALTH PROMOTION

Health promotion is the process of educating others about healthy practices and then supporting those practices among patient populations. Health promotion may be endorsed through such activities as campaigns, individual learning sessions, or media. Within the community, there are several measures that are often promoted among patient populations to enhance health, support healthy behaviors, and prevent disease. Examples include immunization compliance, breast self-exams, diet and exercise programs, smoking-cessation courses, health and safety promotions, nutritional information, stress-management programs, or promotion of the role of religious or spiritual measures into health and wellness.

HEALTHY BEHAVIORS

Healthy behaviors can be addressed at several levels; each level affects and supports the next to promote change and support current interventions for healthy living.

- At the **individual level**, healthy behaviors are addressed by self-examination of healthy practices; setting goals for wellness, such as eating right or engaging in exercise; or attending classes or group meetings that promote healthy activities, such as smoking-cessation classes or stress-management instruction.
- At the **interpersonal group level**, small groups of people gather together to discuss their ideas for healthy behaviors and incorporate them for change. Examples might be walking groups, book clubs that read about healthy living and eating, or weight-loss support groups.
- The **organizational level** encompasses larger groups, such as health care centers, schools, or businesses. These groups support healthy living through campaigns or educational offerings designed to teach those who desire to learn more about healthy practices.

PROMOTING PATIENT ENGAGEMENT

Patients who are actively **engaged** in health promotion and disease prevention tend to have improved outcomes at lower overall cost, so taking steps to engage patients is critical. Patients who are engaged feel more in control of their health care and have an improved experience, making them more likely to have lower rates of out-migration. Patients who have access to their medical records, such as through an online portal, tend to be more engaged and experience greater satisfaction with medical care. Interventions to promote engagement include:

- Develop goals and objectives regarding engagement.
- Utilize appropriate social media and technology such as patient portals, Facebook pages, website, instant messaging, emails, tweets.
- Allow patient interaction with records and staff members via social media/patient portal.
- Provide adequate information/education to improve health literacy.
- Encourage patients to collaborate and make informed decisions.
- Survey patients to ask their opinions and to assess their perceptions of the quality of care.

PROMOTING HEALTHY LIFESTYLES

Because of increased rates of obesity and illnesses associated with unhealthy lifestyles, many nurses are in positions to provide health education and promotion of healthy living practices. Nurses engaging in this type of promotion may help patients to recognize their current weight and set goals for target weights. They may provide education about nutrition or consult with a dietitian who can develop a plan of healthy eating. Nurses may also promote increased activity levels and help patients come up with plans of exercise that will benefit their health. Other programs, such as smoking cessation, management of chronic diseases, safety measures, or stress management may also be incorporated into group-teaching practices to attempt to reach several people at once.

RESILIENCE

Resiliency is a person's ability to adapt to situations when things go wrong. Among patients, resiliency might indicate a response to health care setbacks, complications, or critical diagnoses. Nurses can help patients to develop greater resiliency in the face of health events by encouraging positive behaviors. After talking with patients about their situations, nurses may encourage them to discuss their situations with family or friends who are supportive. Nurses should instill a sense of hope, regardless of the potential outcome, even if the goals are not exactly as patients would wish. It is important for nurses to continue to provide excellent patient care, which reminds patients that they are valued. Finally, patients may need mental health resources if they truly cannot cope with certain situations, and nurses may be able provide references or guidance about getting additional help.

MODIFYING RISK FACTORS

Interventions to **modify risk factors** and promote a healthy lifestyle include:

- Assessing risk factors in all patients and following up at subsequent visits.
- Establishing a baseline for the individual patient by which to measure progress.
- Educating the patient and family about what constitutes risk factors and how these risk factors affect health.
- Counseling patient and assessing the level of motivation for change.
- Educating the patient and family about methods of mitigating risk factors.
- Helping the patient to develop a plan for change.
- Advising patient about community resources available to help reduce risk factors.
- Providing easy access to programs, such as smoking cessation and alcohol rehabilitation, that patients can utilize.
- Tracking patient's program and providing ongoing feedback.

- Developing a reward system to promote adherence.
- Engaging family and friends in helping the patient, such as by joining in exercise regimens or changing diet.
- Developing a plan for maintenance.

HEALTH INTERVENTIONS DIFFERENCES

Nursing interventions are a core component of nursing care, but interventions differ, depending on the population. Nurses who work in acute-care settings have different interventions for patient care than those who work in community-based settings, but there may be some interventions that overlap between the two settings. Clinical nurse leaders determine which interventions are appropriate, depending on the populations they serve. Interventions, such as advocating for patient needs, patient education about the disease processes, and administration of medications may span both the individual and the community interventions. Interventions, such as data analysis of disease surveillance, may be used more often in the community setting compared to acute interventions, such as increasing activity levels, wound irrigation, or checking vital signs, which are applicable to individuals.

STEPS IN DEVELOPING HEALTH PROMOTION PROGRAMS

Steps in developing **health promotion programs** for patient populations include:

1. Identify the target population (adults, elderly, children, neonates).
2. Facilitate input from the population to promote engagement and cooperation and to assist with planning to meet needs.
3. Identify leading health indicators for the population (hypertension, use of tobacco, inactivity, alcohol use, poor diet).
4. Identify and engage partners within the community, such as agencies/organizations, employers, service organizations, faith-based programs, public health agencies, and health care providers.
5. Identify resources to pay for costs associated with interventions, such as grants, budget items, and donations.
6. Develop measurable short-term and long-term goals and objectives.
7. Determine appropriate interventions (screening, education, smoking-cessation programs).
8. Develop a plan and timeframe for implementation of interventions.
9. Begin implementation.
10. Assess implementation, including the percentage of population reached and the rates of participation.
11. Assess achievement of short-term goals to determine effectiveness of interventions.
12. Carry out modifications of plan as needed.
13. Assess long-term goals/outcomes.

COMMUNITY EDUCATION

Community health nurses play important roles in providing education and reducing barriers that may affect access to care. Clinical nurse leaders who work in the community may analyze health trends to determine compliance in healthy activities among some populations. They may organize classes or educational seminars that are accessible to the community and convenient to attend to provide teaching about certain topics that are important to the population. Nurses may help people to organize their care in health centers by attending appointments or follow-up meetings. Finally, community health nurses may develop campaigns against certain practices that are detrimental to the health of the population, may educate community members about the issues, and may give examples for management and prevention.

HEALTH AND WELL-BEING OF OLDER ADULTS

Some nurse leaders are able to partner with providers in the community to support the health and well-being of certain populations, such as older adults. Depending on the area of need, nurses can work with certain groups to provide services for older adults in the community, including immunizations and blood pressure screenings to support health; advice and guidance about nutrition through helping to plan diets; help with mobility and physical access to resources, such as shopping or driving; assistance with medications, including education about dosages and side effects; help with obtaining medical devices ordered by physicians, such as diabetic supplies, mobility devices, or orthopedic resources; and partnership with counselors or therapists to assist some older adults in the community with mental health issues.

LET'S MOVE! CAMPAIGN

The **Let's Move! campaign** was the idea of Michelle Obama as a program designed to target and reduce childhood obesity. The initiative recognizes the propensity for obesity among certain populations and seeks to address contributing factors. The Let's Move! campaign focuses on such activities as providing resources for health and wellness among young children and their families, helping parents and those caring for young children to make choices that will positively affect the health of their children, promoting exercise and increased amounts of physical activity among children, helping schools to design menus that provide healthy foods, and helping people to be able to find and buy health foods for their families.

HEALTHY PEOPLE 2020 INITIATIVE

The **Healthy People 2020** initiative is a campaign that sets objectives for the health of people in America. It is based on scientific methods and is updated every 10 years. The initiative sets many goals for the health of Americans. Its goal for social determinants of health is to design and maintain environments that promote good health to all people. This is done by assessing current environments to determine their health effects, by describing the roles of those involved with improving the health of environments, and by working with organizations and legislators to implement changes that improve environments to promote good public health.

HEALTH CARE SERVICES ACCESS

Nurses may need to help some patients to overcome barriers to finding adequate health care. Some people may find that staying with one health care provider is quite a challenge. Nurses can help to reduce some of the barriers by educating patients about the importance of having a medical home with a knowledgeable physician; by helping patients to call physicians' offices or fill out paperwork for appointments; by providing information and education about medical costs, cost-reduction strategies, or providers who accept Medicare or Medicaid; by helping patients contact physicians who provide culturally appropriate services; and by following up with patients to evaluate any other areas where they might need assistance.

COMMUNITY PARTNERSHIPS

Once risks have been identified and a health promotion program initiated to eliminate or decrease risks, **community partnerships** are essential to successful implementation of the program and attainment of positive outcomes. The first step in establishing community partnerships is to determine which community resources may have a direct involvement or a vested interest in the target population because they may provide invaluable input and services. For example, if the target population is heroin users, community partners that provide services or come in contact with the population may include shelters, Salvation Army®, 12-step programs, police departments, mental health providers, rehabilitation facilities, schools, religious and/or cultural organizations, and physicians. Community organizations that have a vested interest in decreasing heroin use because of community impact may include the Chamber of Commerce, local businesses, and property management organizations. Rarely does one outreach program reach all members of a population, so engaging community partners can multiply opportunities for engagement.

Healthcare Policy

HEALTH CARE BILLS

Because nurses should understand and become involved in the **legislative process** of health care policy and reform, it is important for nurses to first understand the process of how a health care bill eventually becomes law. Initially, an idea for a health care bill is presented, which is introduced to either the Senate or the House. The bill is reviewed by a legislative representative who determines whether it is appropriate. The bill is then read before either the House or the Senate committee. After reading, the bill is then presented to the opposite committee for approval. For example, if a bill is read before the House, it must then be read before the Senate, as a bill must be approved by both the House and the Senate before it can move forward. Finally, when the bill is approved, it becomes a law after it is signed by the president.

HEALTH POLICY

According to the World Health Organization, **health policy** refers to "decisions, plans, and actions . . . to achieve specific health care goals within a society." Health policy is utilized to make future plans for the direction of health care and to serve as a guide to researchers and health care professionals. Health policy may be worldwide (preventing pandemics) as with programs of the United Nations and WHO, national (decreasing neonatal deaths, rates of HIV infections), local (decreasing lead exposure, improving air quality), or organizational (improving quality of care, carrying out lobbying activities). A health policy should clearly communicate goals as well as roles and responsibilities for achieving these goals. Health policy often includes targets as well as a timeline for achieving those targets. Major health policies include *Healthy People 2020* in the United States and *Health 2020*, the European health policy. Both health policies set specific health priorities.

REGULATORY CONTROLS

Regulatory controls are limits and requirements health care organizations must follow that ensure they are in line with the standards set by the regulatory agency. Regulatory agencies monitor compliance of hospitals and health care centers with set standards. Examples of regulatory agencies include the US Food and Drug Administration or the Centers for Medicare and Medicaid Services. These controls go hand-in-hand with quality-assurance activities because they are designed to set standards that promote safety, make changes, or provide payment for services for patients. Quality provides a sense of satisfaction from the patients, and providing safe care in an environment that complies with regulatory objectives sustains quality assurance.

AMERICAN RECOVERY AND REINVESTMENT ACT

The **American Recovery and Reinvestment Act** (Recovery Act) was passed in 2009 with the goals of supporting jobs, encouraging economic activity, and requiring accountability for government spending. The Recovery Act designated money to be spent on public health programs, specifically public health and prevention campaigns to increase preventive care, with the goal of ultimately reducing spending on treatment and management of acute and chronic conditions. Another aspect of the Recovery Act was to spend more money on health care technology designed to improve communication among providers and provide access to more evidence-based practice guidelines.

ELECTRONIC HEALTH RECORDS STANDARDS

The American Recovery and Reinvestment Act of 2009 designated money to help providers and hospitals to implement **electronic health records (EHR).** With this comes the increase in EHRs as methods of tracking and documenting patient care. However, when patients are seen at more than one health care organization, the EHRs may or may not be compatible. This limits the ability to send information between locations and decreases communication, potentially leading to errors, missed reports, and repeated procedures. Electronic health records must have standards set by using the same or compatible software programs to send and receive information between providers. Additionally, changing from paper charts to EHRs is a potentially cumbersome process that might involve loss of essential information if not performed correctly. Standards must be set and followed to acquire the benefits associated with EHRs.

COST-CONTAINMENT

Nurses are often put in difficult situations when policies that are focused on **cost-containment** direct their efforts at patient care. When nurses work under regulatory agencies that pay for patient care, they provide only certain services for which they are paid. However, some patients need additional services than what is covered but cannot receive them because of cost-containment policies. Nurses can work against some of these restrictions by becoming involved with legislative decisions and speaking with decision-makers about the effects of restrictions on patient care. Additionally, nurses can educate politicians and lawmakers about the necessity of certain types of patient care and their limitations due to health policies. Finally, nurses can form groups that will work together to provide education, position statements, petitions, and opportunities for public speaking to get the word out about the importance of change in particular areas.

MANDATING EMPLOYER-BASED FINANCING DISADVANTAGES

In the United States, an ideal health coverage system is one in which employers provide insurance for their employees as part of the benefits package offered by the company. However, many people change jobs and do not stay with one employer long enough to derive benefits. Additionally, some people might stay only for the health insurance coverage or to avoid gaps in coverage. Employers might have difficulty accessing policies that are affordable to both them and to employees, and some premiums are extremely high, even with employer-based contributions. Additionally, even with employers financing some of the costs of premiums for health insurance, patients often still must pay large co-payments or co-insurance. Finally, there are still many people who remain unemployed, who have no coverage, which leaves those with jobs paying increased costs to cover payments for the uninsured.

CHILDREN'S HEALTH INSURANCE PROGRAM

The **Children's Health Insurance Program (CHIP)** was created in 1997 and was designed to provide health coverage for families with children who do not have insurance or who meet low-income guidelines. CHIP is governed by each state, but part of its financing comes from the federal government. Each state has guidelines for eligibility, the amount of coverage provided, and specific policies. CHIP covers care for children in hospitals, outpatient programs, and emergency care. This includes well-child visits and immunizations. These provisions are allowed by all states, and then there are some states that provide further coverage, such as mental health coverage and substance abuse treatment.

IMPLEMENTING POLICIES FOR PREVENTIVE CARE

While preventive care has been shown to benefit Americans, to reduce the severity of chronic disease, and to promote health and wellness, there are some opponents to increased spending on preventive care. To pass health policy into action often requires more money directed at certain programs at which the policy is directed. For some, increasing spending on preventive care is not a good idea because they believe that people will not change their behaviors, even with increased campaigns. Additionally, many people argue that health care workers today are trained for treating and managing disease, not preventing it. It would take more money to prevent disease and to train providers in preventive care. The payments for health care spending are also focused on acute and chronic management of illness in health care organizations. If preventive care must be supported financially, it would take a large amount of time, effort, and money to restructure the reimbursement process to pay for such measures.

LITERATURE RELATED TO HEALTH POLICY

Health policy information may be available in numerous locations, such as organizational briefs, news reports, and websites. Many nurses do not have the time to perform thorough searches for policy information and need to find methods of accessing accurate information quickly. Nurses should begin by asking themselves what information they need by constructing a question about the topic. They then can take the broad points from the question to implement into a search for information. Using key phrases from their thoughts or questions, nurses can search for information, using databases or the internet to find health policy literature related to their topic. It is important to keep information concise when searching to avoid getting too many results that would require too much time to research. Some computerized databases use Boolean logic, which helps to organize information by creating combinations of concepts that can be searched, which narrows the field of results.

HEALTH POLICY INFORMATION EVALUATION

Nurses who are searching for health policy information may come upon sources, which are accurate and reflective, but others that are outdated or even erroneous. It is important to **evaluate information** carefully to ensure that it is accurate and up-to-date. When accessing information, nurse should consider the source of the documents and whether or not they have references. When searching the internet, nurses should check the reliability of the website. Nurses should obtain information that is unbiased and controlled, rather than spending time reading opinions, blogs, or personal views that might have political agendas. The information should be relatively current to be accurate. Finally, the information should be organized in such a manner that it is easily searchable and relatively easy to read. Taking time to define certain words or concepts because data are presented in complex jargon will make the process more difficult, and nurses may be less likely to follow through if this is the case.

IMPACT OF HEALTH IN THE GLOBAL ENVIRONMENT

Despite advances in medicine and nursing care in the United States and other developed countries, mortality rates are high. Increased care of patients from developing countries because of immigration as well as recruitment of nursing staff from developing countries can affect the work of nursing staff in the United States. More and more, nurses are caring for patients who not only have language barriers and different cultural backgrounds but who may have been in the United States only for a brief period of time before seeking health care. These patients often have a high incidence of illnesses that are endemic to their countries. They may have little experience in the health care environment of the United States or with even seeking health care at all. Nurses need to be prepared to face cultural issues as well as potentially new behaviors, languages, illnesses, and expectations from patients who come to the United States and who need health care.

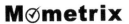

IMPACT OF HEALTH CARE POLICY

Health care policy impacts:

- **Health promotion/Disease prevention**: Health care policy affects the allocation of funds for health promotion/disease prevention at national, state, and local levels, and health care policy may be influenced by politics. For example, under conservative health care policies, sex education for minors focused on abstinence despite studies showing it to be an unsuccessful approach, and funding for birth control was cut.
- **Standards of care**: Health care policy may focus on carrying out specific interventions (such as giving aspirin to patients experiencing a possible heart attack) and outcomes (duration of stay), requiring a change in the standards of care in order to carry out the policies.
- **Scope of practice**: The professional's scope of practice is determined at the state level but may be influenced by national standards and different approaches to health care policy. For example, prescriptive authority may change.
- **Access to care**: Health care policy, which can include financing systems, can either increase access to care (such as the Affordable Care Act) or decrease access (Medicaid cutbacks).

APPLIED HEALTH POLICY DIRECTIVES

Health policy directives are instructions given about how to implement health practices that have been passed by legislation. In many cases, health policy directives consider current health situations and set goals or specific guidelines accordingly. Nursing research often responds to health policy directives by using the information available through the policy to ask questions about how they affect nursing research, what interventions can be changed that support the directives, or how the nursing profession can respond to the directives. Once a topic is selected, nursing research focuses on answering the specific question. The results of the research can then be applied to practice, as well as support the directives if the outcomes are applicable.

Care Environment Management

Knowledge Management

KNOWLEDGE IN CARE MANAGEMENT

Knowledge is having an understanding of certain concepts; knowing information is critical to providing care for patients, yet patients must also develop certain levels of knowing to understand their own condition and care requirements. There are different types of knowing, each of which may offer a greater understanding of how a person knows things.

- **Personal knowing** involves how nurses understand themselves and their own views, beliefs, and knowledge. Personal knowing may also describe how the relationship between patients and nurses develops.
- **Aesthetic knowing** concentrates on how nurses perceive patients and their needs, as well as those aspects of the relationship that are distinctive or unique.
- **Ethical knowing** is the understanding of what is moral or ethical, such as nurses' knowledge of measures that are correct in behavior, policies, and actions.

INTERDISCIPLINARY RESEARCH

Interdisciplinary research involves multiple disciplines working together to perform research, the results of which may then be put into clinical practice. Because health care is becoming increasingly complex, requiring the services of multiple professions for adequate care, interdisciplinary research focuses on the total care of the population, using perspectives from various disciplines. The interdisciplinary research team has the capability to respond to complex dilemmas that are questioned and sorted through research. Nurses are in a position to lead the interdisciplinary team because nursing includes a background in a number of different disciplines. For example, nursing students may practice in various areas, including physical or occupational therapy, nutrition, or social services. Because these areas are often incorporated into nursing practice, nurses may hold greater knowledge, making them obvious choices for team leaders in interdisciplinary research.

DISEASE SURVEILLANCE

Disease surveillance is the process of collecting data, analyzing it, and implementing new measures in response to a disease that has developed within a population. Disease surveillance is often used by public health officials and public health nurses to discover how diseases develop in communities and to prevent unhealthy outcomes. Data obtained from disease surveillance measures may be used to help public health officials implement systems of prevention, determine which communities are at risk for outbreaks, make changes in policies that protect communities from disease outbreaks, monitor the course of the disease and how it progresses, collect resources for disease treatment and prevention, and create reports of how the disease affects the community.

ROLE OF NURSES IN DISEASE SURVEILLANCE

Nurses who work in **disease surveillance** are responsible for monitoring the outbreak of disease in the community, tracking how it spreads, and determining how it affects the population. The disease outbreaks that nurses trained in surveillance may track include influenza, tick-borne diseases, sexually transmitted diseases, or HIV. Additionally, surveillance nurses may also monitor rates of chronic diseases in the community, such as asthma or diabetes. They gather information from health centers that care for patients with these conditions, as well as other sources of reported

72

data, such as schools or child-care centers. Surveillance nurses must be able to understand clinical research and statistics and may be responsible for performing research studies or providing statistical data.

DATA SETS

Data sets are comprised of information applied to statistical analysis that is then investigated as part of disease surveillance. Nurses who play a role in epidemiology use data sets to analyze and interpret information to determine outcomes, such as how disease affects communities or how specific diseases are spread within populations. Data sets come from facts about the situation being analyzed; for example, a data set about malaria may come from the World Health Organization, current population descriptions, or clinical trials. Each data set has several factors, or variables, that make up the set to be used. Using the malaria example, the nurse identifying information for the data set may separate it into variables, such as how many cases have been reported in the last year, the date of the first reported case, and the number of deaths reported.

QUANTITATIVE AND QUALITATIVE DATA

Quantitative data comprise information that can be directly measured. In research, quantitative data are those that provide cause and effect outcomes with hard facts that are represented by statistical analysis. An example of quantitative research is as follows: if nurses working in an intensive care unit want to develop procedures to protect against infection, they must first determine how often patients develop ventilator-associated pneumonia within a given time period. The results would be numbers that they can directly measure over time.

Qualitative analysis involves research that is difficult to measure in terms of actual numerical data. These data are subjective; they may lend to theory development, and the results are often written out descriptively rather than numerically. An example of qualitative nursing research might be examining nurses' responses to changes in policy regarding the handoffs of patients. The outcomes are subjective and based on the opinions of nurses, which cannot be reported numerically.

SCIENTIFIC METHOD

The **scientific method** is used in science to ask questions about a particular situation, analyze the information, and perform experiments to find answers. The scientific method is not entirely unlike the nursing process in that the nursing process also seeks to find answers about a situation, usually patient care. The scientific method starts with defining the problem and collecting data about the problem. This is similar to the first step of the nursing process, which is patient assessment, which identifies the patient's problem and contributing factors. The next portion of the scientific method is formulating a hypothesis, while the next steps of the nursing process are formulating a nursing diagnosis and identifying outcomes. The scientific method then plans for testing the hypothesis and then takes steps to test it. Similarly, the nursing process plans for patient care and then implements interventions to achieve identified outcomes. The final steps of both the scientific method and the nursing process are to evaluate the methods to determine effectiveness.

BENCHMARKING

Benchmarking is when nurses compare standards, policies, and practices in an organization with those of other health care centers to determine where changes can be made to improve practice. Benchmarking might take place in quality-improvement areas to best determine patient-safety measures; it might also be used to explain the need for further resources, to reflect on current practices to determine successes and failures; to make changes in care practices, such as handoffs of patients by nurses, medication administration, or infection control; and to improve communication among the members of the interdisciplinary team.

GAINING INFORMATION FOR COMPARISONS

Nurses who perform benchmarking comparisons may gain their information in a variety of ways. They may perform literature reviews of practice results from other organizations and compare statistical data. They may read best-practice articles written by members of organizations that have implemented new practices successfully. Nurses may also meet with teams from other organizations to compare practices and develop new measures, if necessary. In some situations, nurses may also meet with others through seminars, educational offerings, forums, or community meetings to compare and contrast practices and determine where changes can be made.

ACCOUNTABILITY AND RESPONSIBILITY

While similar in scope of practice, **nursing accountability** in the workplace differs from the responsibilities of the nurse. Nursing accountability refers to the willingness of nurses to act in a trustworthy manner and accept the outcomes of their behavior, understanding that they are responsible for their own behavior.

Alternatively, **responsibility** describes this process of action, in which nurses behave in a way that is trustworthy, credible, and dependable. Nurses who practice accountability provide autonomy for patients to make their own decisions while guiding them in a responsible manner. The nurses not only have the authority to act in this manner, it is their obligation as part of the profession.

ACCOUNTABILITY

Professional nurses are accountable to various population groups with whom they work. In practice with patients, nurses have a duty to provide safe patient care that minimizes risks. They must demonstrate clinical competency that gives their patients and their colleague's confidence in their abilities as clinicians. Nurses must respect the differences in beliefs and practices of both their coworkers and their patients, treating others with dignity. Among personnel, nurses use strategies to resolve conflict as well as to share pertinent information while preserving the privacy of patients. Finally, nurses serve as advocates for both their patients and the nursing profession as a whole to ensure patients get the care that they need and to promote respect for all nurses.

NURSING ACCOUNTABILITY

Nursing accountability involves various **components** that must be upheld to provide committed care in which nurses take responsibility for their actions.

- **Clarity** involves understanding what the expectations are of nurses in each situation so that they know their duties and can fulfill their role.
- **Outcomes** are potentially positive or negative consequences that may occur when nurses hold themselves accountable. Despite the potential for negative outcomes, nurses must uphold their own accountability in practice as an ethical responsibility and to prevent future negative outcomes, if at all possible.
- **Commitment** is the nurses' obligation to keep themselves accountable for their actions. Commitment means nurses already understand the goals of their work and vow to complete their tasks in a responsible and appropriate way.

ENCOURAGING ACCOUNTABILITY

All nurses must be accountable for their actions. It may be helpful to think of accountability as a chain, in that each nurse serves as a link to provide exceptional and responsible care. Clinical nurse leaders can **promote accountability** among their staff and maintain the chain of accountability by acting as leaders who are trustworthy to others. This may encourage nurses to seek clinical nurse leaders as resources or guides for their actions. They may also motivate other nurses to remain accountable by providing options for education or team-building exercises. Part of the role of clinical nurse leaders is to inform other nurses about their levels of accountability: what is acceptable and what needs to be cultivated. Finally, clinical nurse leaders can foster accountability with others by being consistent in their own behaviors and by showing accountability to their patients as well as to the nurses with whom they work.

Healthcare Systems/Organizations

HEALTH CARE FINANCING SYSTEMS

Health care financing systems include:

- **Beveridge Model:** Developed by William Beveridge for the National Health Service in the UK. With this system, citizens have a health card that gives them access to health care for which the government pays through taxes, so users do not receive bills for service. There are both government-owned hospitals with employed physicians, and private providers, but the private providers bill the government directly for services. The government sets prices and fees to keep costs low. This model is in also in use in Scandinavia.
- **Bismarck Model:** All citizens are covered by insurance ("sickness funds") with costs of insurance paid for by both employers and employees. This model was envisioned as a right of labor, aimed at the employed. Costs are contained as insurance companies are precluded from making a profit. Most health care providers are privately contracted. This model is in use in Germany, France, and Japan and other countries.
- **National Health Insurance Model**: Developed in Canada as a single-payer system with the government funding the insurance program; however, some services are not covered or are limited and waits may be required for some treatments, so many people opt for supplementary insurance policies. However, this type of single-payer system provides leverage for negotiation, so costs may be contained.
- **Out-of-Pocket Model**: People required to pay out-of-pocket for health care services because they do not have insurance or government provided medical assistance (such as Medicaid). In some countries, people barter for services, but in the United States, people may incur huge medical bills or simply go without necessary care and treatment because they lack adequate income to pay for health care services. Free clinics and some faith-based programs may provide some services for those who cannot pay.

UNIVERSAL HEALTH CARE MODEL

With the **universal health care model**, a system of health care financing is in place in which all citizens receive a health card that provides them access to care at no additional cost or limited additional cost. In some countries, universal health is paid for by taxes through a single payer system, while other systems are paid for from both public and private sources (such as from employers). Some systems require that all citizens purchase health coverage (generally with subsidies provided for those with low income), similar to the program instituted under the Affordable Care Act. A universal health care model usually covers all basic care and services, but citizens may need supplementary insurance for other services, such as medications or mental health care. The primary goals of the universal health care model are to improve health outcomes for citizens and reduce costs by pooling financial risks and improving general health through increased access to care.

PUBLIC HEALTH

Public health is a system of practice that typically takes place within the community as opposed to the health care organization. Public health is focused on preventing disease through education, policies, and campaigns. While many inpatient health care organizations are associated with treating and managing disease, public health seeks to prevent many diseases before they develop. Public health and inpatient care are connected within health care, as patients who seek inpatient services may need ongoing public health care after dismissal. Education can be provided within the inpatient setting that promotes a healthy lifestyle and prevention of disease and further complications. Patients who use public health nursing services may continue to be monitored by these nurses while in the hospital; when released, these patients continue with their public health nurses after discharge.

OUTCOMES MEASURED BY HEALTH CARE SYSTEMS

Patient outcomes may be measured to determine the impact of nursing interventions at the clinical level. **Health care organizations** may also measure outcomes that determine how well resources are used. Some outcomes that health care organizations may measure include the types of nurses available to provide care, such as registered nurses or advanced-practice nurses; the setting where care is provided, including the hospital, clinic, long-term care facility, or home; the population of patients affected, such as those requiring acute care or those needing long-term care; and the cultures affected, including those with language barriers, those with various cultural practices, and those with diverse religious beliefs.

HEALTH CARE SYSTEM'S RESPONSE TO CHANGE

Change is occurring within health care systems all the time, whether it is recognized or not. Health care systems may encounter resistance when changes are applied within the health care setting. It is important for nurses to understand reasons for resistance to change so that they can work to either counteract the resistance or ensure that change becomes acceptable. How the information about the change is perceived has an effect on how it is accepted; it is often affected by how the change is presented. Openness to change is affected by the perceived roles of those involved in the change. Response to change is also affected by who is involved with planning and creating the change. When those who need to change are involved in the process of making the change, there may be less opposition.

FACTORS THAT INFLUENCE HEALTH CARE DELIVERY

The **delivery of care** is impacted by various factors:

- **Political forces** affect medical care as the Federal and state governments increasingly become purchasers of medical care, imposing their guidelines and limitations on the medical system. A change in leadership, especially at the national level, may limit or expand insurance and Medicaid coverage.
- **Regulatory/Legal forces** may be local, state, or Federal and can have a profound effect of delivery of care and services, differing from one state or region to another. CMS, for example, often guides insurance practice; so, for example, if Medicare does not cover a type of care, insurance companies also refuse coverage.
- **Economic forces**, such as managed care or cost-containment committees, try to contain costs to insurers and facilities by controlling access to and duration of treatment, and limiting products. Economic pressure is working to prevent duplication of services in a geographical area, and providers are creating networks to purchase supplies and equipment directly.

Interprofessional Communication

ASSERTIVE COMMUNICATION TECHNIQUES

While working on the interdisciplinary team, nurses may need to employ certain communication techniques to avoid misunderstandings and to send clear messages. Because several disciplines may be working together on a team, it is important to use effective communication to understand fully the role of each team member.

Assertive communication gets the point across without being too aggressive. When using assertive communication, nurses should use statements that start with "I...," which are much less threatening than starting phrases with "You...," which sounds accusatory and may increase the likelihood of a defensive reaction. Nurses should also acknowledge the other person's position by making a statement of understanding before launching into their own explanation. Finally, if nurses do not have an immediate solution to a problem, they should determine what they could do to solve the problem by working together with others.

DIALOGUE, APPRECIATIVE INQUIRY AND OBSERVATION

In the group setting, nurse leaders can garner plenty of information and understanding about those with whom they work.

- **Dialogue** is the process of conversing with others to share background assumptions, values, and ideas. Dialogue also allows nurses to clarify points of potential miscommunication. This form of communication is done deliberately to facilitate better understanding between team members.
- **Appreciative inquiry** focuses on the strengths of those on the team and the potential outcomes of the work of the team. This approach involves facilitating a vision for the group and allows group members to brainstorm about ideas or goals for the group.
- **Observation** involves listening to and watching the behavior of other team members to better understand their point of view. Observation is more about listening and less about talking, avoiding interruptions that may affect communication.

SBAR

The **SBAR** acronym is used when communicating information, typically to a provider. The SBAR provides a guide for how to present information that is clear and structured and allows nurses to get to the point, rather than rambling about extraneous information.

- The S in SBAR stands for **situation**, in which nurses explain the current situation and reason for contact.
- The B stands for **background**. Nurses give pertinent background information that is related to the situation described, including important medical history and the results of treatments or laboratory work.
- The A stands for **assessment**, in which nurses compare the situation and the patient's background with the current clinical picture and the data gained from the nursing assessment.
- The R stands for **recommendation**, in which nurses and providers discuss what is needed next to manage the situation.

REPORTING CHANGES

Important aspects of caring for patients include providing appropriate and safe care and monitoring for changes in the condition of patients. However, it is not enough to just monitor their condition; nurses must also **report changes** that occur to uphold safety and to continue timely and appropriate care. If there are changes, nurses have a duty to report the changes to providers so that they are aware of the situation and may possibly provide orders for what is to be done to manage the situation. Nurses are liable if they do not report changes that may involve deterioration of a medical condition; legal action can be taken against nurses if they fail to respond.

OBJECTIVE DATA AND SUBJECTIVE DATA

When communicating and documenting information about patients, nurses may use either objective data or subjective data.

- **Objective data** are observable, based on facts, and can be measured. Examples of objective data include patients' vital signs, medications administered, intake and output, or illness symptoms that are observed, such as skin changes, cyanosis, perspiration, tremor, or vomiting.
- Alternatively, **subjective data** convey information nurses receive from patients. Subjective information can be gained through patients' interviews, patients' descriptions of how they feel, descriptions of symptoms they feel that are not necessarily evident, such as nausea, and information about their beliefs and preferences.

PHONE ORDERS

Telephone orders from physicians may reduce the time it takes for nurses to get results for patient care, but phone orders may also increase the risk of errors. When taking orders over the phone from physicians, nurses should always speak directly to the physician, rather than documenting orders from a third party. The order should be written exactly as the physician gave it, noting the date and time of the order and stating that it was taken over the phone. Nurses must then write the names of the physician giving the orders and then sign their own name afterward. After orders are taken, nurses should repeat them back to the physician to ensure they received the correct information and to clarify any misconceptions. When documenting the order, nurses then document that it was read back to the physician, which is a stated communication goal of the Joint Commission.

COMMUNICATING CRITICAL RESULTS

Communication of critical results in a timely manner is one of the National Patient Safety Goals created by the Joint Commission. The goal considers the timely action of communicating critical results of laboratory tests or diagnostic procedures by providers. Failure to report in a timely manner can cause significant patient complications and could lead to life-threatening consequences. The Joint Commission recommends devising policies that give parameters for what results are considered critical and for developing appropriate timeframes for communication. This practice ultimately improves communication among providers when it is carried out sufficiently, so that nurses and physicians work together to provide patient care, respond to changes, and prevent the deterioration of their patients.

IMPROVING COMMUNICATION

One of the roles of clinical nurse leaders is to **reduce communication gaps**, which can cause fragmented patient care. Clinical nurse leaders are responsible for improving communication, both between nursing staff and between nurses and physicians. This may involve assessing nursing report styles and evaluating the effectiveness of handoffs. Clinical nurse leaders may need to develop systems of giving and receiving reports between providers that are effective and cover pertinent information about patients. Additionally, clinical nurse leaders may need to develop a communication system among nurses who have previously cared for the patient and who need to pass along information, depending on the health care unit's approach to nursing care. Clinical nurse leaders may become liaisons between staff nurses and physicians. This involves developing positive professional relationships with physicians to bridge the gap between the nursing staff and medical staff.

HOSPITALIST

Hospitalists are physicians who specifically care for patients in the hospital. These physicians often have a background in internal medicine. Hospitalists are available in the hospital to meet with staff regarding patients' conditions, to diagnose and provide orders for treatment, and to provide instruction and guidance directly to hospitalized patients. Clinical nurse leaders who work in hospitals interact with hospitalists regularly. Clinical nurse leaders may act as liaisons between nursing staff and hospitalists to help direct efforts for care as it passes from orders to implementation. The role of hospitalists was developed to assist with the duties of primary care physicians by reducing time they spent going back and forth between their offices and the hospital and to provide specialized care from physicians who are dedicated to the specific needs of hospitalized patients.

DISSEMINATING INFORMATION BARRIERS

When presenting information to other professionals or the interdisciplinary team, nurses may encounter several **barriers** related to their own limitations or the capacities for others to absorb such information. Nurses may doubt their own abilities to present information, citing poor communication skills or anxiety. They may not have time to put the information together in a way that can be presented professionally, such as taking the time to write an article or develop a short presentation. Nurses may not know what to do to begin when they are developing information to present to others and so may not even get started. Finally, nurses may fear criticism of their work, which blocks them from taking steps to present to avoid the analysis or critical assessment of their presentations.

EFFECTIVE COMMUNICATION

Effective communication between disciplines is often **challenging** because of the dynamics of different groups. Each discipline has its own priorities, some of which may be very different, for what patients need. Often, each discipline focuses on its own goals, and sometimes the objectives of other team members may compete for top priority. Gaps in communication may develop because of proximity; if team members work at various locations or there are difficulties with scheduling or attending meetings, important information may fall through the cracks. Some nurses may feel a distance between their profession and that of physicians, which may make communication difficult. Disciplines that require various skill mixes or different levels of education may create gaps in communication as a result of a lack of understanding of the work requirements of others.

NEGOTIATION SKILLS

Almost all interprofessional communication and collaboration requires **negotiation** in order to reach consensus because participants bring various perspectives and may have different needs and motivations. Negotiation skills include the ability to:

- Listen actively and provide feedback.
- Outline needs and responsibilities and understand cause and effect.
- Research and present data and predict outcomes based on data.
- Deal with facts rather than emotions.
- Prioritize issues.
- Utilize various bargaining strategies:

- o Distributive: A competitive process in which one side wins and the other loses (zero-sum, win-lose). May lead to compromise or stalemate.
- o Integrative: A collaborative process (win-win). The parties involved bargain jointly, trying to solve problems. Integrative bargaining is most successful if the parties have developed trust.
- o Mixed: Combines some aspects of distributive and integrative.
- Understand conflict resolution strategies: accommodating, avoiding, collaborating, competing, compromising, confronting, forcing, negotiating, reassuring, problem-solving, and withdrawing.

Teamwork

INTERDISCIPLINARY HEALTH CARE TEAM FUNCTIONS

Regardless of the reasons for a team meeting, there are several common **functions** shared by most, whether the team is meeting to discuss patient care or to perform other duties, such as developing a new educational curriculum. Teams share common goals in that they meet together for a purpose. The team members each have their roles and should identify their positions for contributing to the goals of the team. Members of the team are often included because they have something specific to share; for example, an interdisciplinary team made up of professionals discussing patient-care management might consist of a physical therapist, a nurse, and a physician, as each of these roles brings expertise in their own areas. The team's purpose is to have an action; the team ultimately has a purpose for meeting and pursues that purpose to meet a goal.

ROLES ON AN INTERDISCIPLINARY TEAM

There may be several different disciplines engaged in patient care as part of an **interdisciplinary team**. Some examples of team members include physicians, social service workers, pharmacists, nutritionists, physical or occupational therapists, or mental health practitioners. Most professions overlap with nursing in some way, as nurses often provide comprehensive care that may touch on the work of different disciplines. Nurses provide medication and treatments as ordered by physicians and pharmacists. They may work in case management to help patients with social services, such as disability care or finding financial assistance. Nurses often give patients their meals and understand how nutrition affects health, which is similar to the work of nutritionists. They may assist patients with ambulation or activities of daily living, which is also incorporated into the work of physical or occupational therapists. They frequently develop therapeutic relationships with patients and care for their mental health in ways similar to what mental health practitioners do.

SUCCESSFUL INTERDISCIPLINARY TEAMS

Functional interdisciplinary teams have several attributes in common, in that they are productive, patient-centered, and organized. Successful interdisciplinary teams are able to plan for what information they need to cover and what must be discussed during meetings. They set reasonable goals that are achievable and then evaluate effectiveness after a period of time. The role of each team member is made clear to all so that each person understands the duties of the others. This improves communication when everyone knows their own roles and to whom to go for information about specific concepts. If specific people have more education, training, or talent in certain areas, they may become resources for the rest of the group. In some groups, one person may become the leader, while in others, group members share leadership. In either case, leadership is clear and effective to promote the objectives of the team.

MAINTAINING WORKING RELATIONSHIPS

Clinical nurse leaders are not only in unique positions to work side by side with staff, but also to guide them in their practices. **Maintaining positive working relationships** means being a leader to staff and displaying those qualities and responses that are appropriate and will build confidence among staff members while supporting a team environment. Nurse leaders are those to whom others look for guidance by establishing their trust in the nurse leaders expertise as a clinician. Nurse leaders also respect the ideas of staff, recognizing their contributions and expertise in the clinical area. Clinical nurse leaders provide ongoing support for clinical work and collaborate on essential issues to help solve problems. They also provide feedback that is constructive, helping staff to reflect on their weaknesses but build on their strengths.

TEAM-BUILDING EXERCISES

As an organizer and guide for staff nurses, clinical nurse leaders often must collaborate with nursing staff but must also build a nursing team, which functions as a competent and professional workforce. Although many nurses are required to work on teams as part of their jobs, nurse leaders can facilitate **team building** so that those involved feel proud to serve with others and confident in their abilities. Some ideas of team-building exercises include having team meetings on a regular basis to keep everyone updated on the working situation, providing educational opportunities for team members to keep up-to-date on their skills, promoting team activities that involve team members working together and having fun at the same time, and recognizing the strengths of team members to find ways that they can best get involved to serve the team through their expertise and talents.

PHASES OF COLLABORATION

The collaboration process is often discussed, but many times, nurse leaders are not educated or prepared to lead groups to help everyone reach their goals for patient care.

1. During the collaboration process, **problem-setting** identifies those people who are present to serve as part of the team, the individual roles as part of the team, and their ideas for what the initial problem is.
2. During the **direction-setting** phase, the team works together to establish the identified problem and discusses what resources are available that can be used toward solving the problem.
3. Finally, during the **structuring phase**, the required actions and responsibilities are divided among team members, according to their professional expertise. Roles are assigned and clarified so that everyone understands their responsibilities of working toward the optimal outcome of the patient.

GROUPTHINK

Groupthink is a concept that occurs when all members of a group hold the same view or position on a matter. Groupthink may be positive in situations where all team members agree, and there is little cause for problems to develop because of disagreements. In many cases, though, groupthink limits the possibilities for discussion, exchange of ideas, or alternatives to current practices. When developing patient-focused care measures, groupthink can limit how processes occur if all members of the team think alike. In this situation, members may consider that "this is the way it has always been done" and may not be willing to make changes that could be positive for patients. Alternatively, groupthink could be a positive force in developing care that is patient-focused if all team members are on the same page about the importance of certain measures, the best ways to improve or maintain positive practices, and the best practices to improve the quality of patient care.

TYPES OF GROUP PROCESSING

Nurses who participate in group processes may recognize that there are different types of groups that serve different purposes and that are organized by purpose and potential outcomes.

- **Task groups** are designed to develop, plan, and implement a certain task. An example of a task group might be a conference planning committee, which is designed to develop, plan, and put on a conference.
- A **teaching group** meets to provide education. An example of a teaching group might be an educational forum for patients so they can learn about exercise and weight control. The teaching group may develop the information for patients as well as teach it to them.
- A **therapeutic group** is designed to manage situations that may cause stress or emotional disturbances. An example of a therapeutic group might be a support group for patients who have lost loved ones to cancer.

ERROR-MAKING PROCESS AND THE ERROR-RECOVERY PROCESS

Groups are required for decision-making regarding many different aspects of nursing care, including education, interdisciplinary patient care, and quality measures. While groups can effectively make decisions, they can also be responsible for errors.

- The **error-making process** occurs when either one person on the team or a group of team members contribute to an error in decision-making. They may have made the error based on incorrect information, poor communication, or issues of opinion. Once an error is made, the error-recovery process is a necessary component of group work in that the error is brought to the attention of team members, and then the team works together to take action to correct it.
- The **error-recovery process** is necessary once an error has been discovered, whether it was the result of an individual or group making the mistake.

LACK OF INTERDISCIPLINARY TEAMWORK

Interdisciplinary teamwork provides comprehensive patient care not only because many disciplines are involved, but also because team members who are responsible for the care of patients are all talking to each other. Without interdisciplinary teamwork, care of patients can become **fragmented** because of a breakdown in communication. Individual disciplines may each develop care plans for patients or may have their own methods of documenting patient care, which may or may not be related to the care given by others. Additionally, patients' goals may be difficult to identify, and steps toward achieving those goals could be duplicated or omitted completely. Finally, a lack of interdisciplinary teamwork leaves out patients' input and their ideas or wishes for their care. Often patients are the best source of information about the next steps to make in treatment, and without this input, care may be delayed or inadequate.

PROCESS OF CONFLICT STAGES

Conflict is a common occurrence among groups of people who must collaborate for certain goals. When it develops, conflict may progress through a series of stages.

- **Differences** occur when members of the group realize that they do not see eye to eye on a certain topic. The people involved give their opinions of the situation.
- **Discord** happens when people realize that their ideas do not match. During this phase, people may take sides on the issue or may begin to become protective toward their own interests in the situation.

- **Dispute** is the stage in which conflict may evolve, but hopefully nurses can intervene and make changes before the situation reaches this point. A dispute occurs when members of the group argue over the conflict. This may cause great tension, defensiveness, or emotional reactions from group members that must be curtailed by considering the different perspectives and establishing a goal to resolve the conflict.

EMOTIONAL CONFLICT AND TASK CONFLICT

When working in a group setting, **conflict** may be inevitable, but learning how to manage conflict is an important role of nurse leaders. Conflict may arise from misunderstandings or miscommunication about activities. Emotional conflict occurs when team members have a personal or emotional basis for their disagreement. It may arise as a result of hurt feelings over a misunderstanding, feelings of inferiority because of attitudes, or because of unresolved task conflicts. Task conflict occurs when team members disagree about certain practices. This may be because of educational differences, diversity in skill levels, or differences of opinion. As a potential group leader, it is important for nurses to understand the different types of conflict, which can then guide them toward better conflict resolution.

AVID

Because conflict is often inevitable within the clinical environment, nurses must be familiar with certain strategies to manage conflict. The **AVID approach** is an acronym that describes a method of communication and response to prevent conflict from escalating.

- The A stands for **assume**, in which nurses assume positive things about those with whom they working.
- The V stands for **validate**, in which nurses listen to another's point of view and confirm their feelings about the situation, even when they do not agree.
- The I stands for **ignore**, which means that if nurses are unable to change a situation or validate it in a meaningful way, they should ignore it and move on.
- The D stands for **do,** as in do something. If assuming the positive, validating another's point of view, and ignoring the situation do not work, nurses must do something to prevent the stress of conflict from negatively affecting them.

POSITIVE ENVIRONMENT

Part of the role of clinical nurse leaders is to assess the culture of the environment in which they work and act as liaisons between staff and management. When staff nurses are unhappy with their work environment, it can result in dissatisfaction among those who are providing frontline care. Clinical nurse leaders can **promote a positive work environment** by recognizing what staff nurses want, such as better scheduled hours, increased pay, or greater bonuses. Clinical nurse leaders may not be able to provide all of these things, but they can improve staff morale by letting them know that their concerns are understood. Clinical nurse leaders can also make an effort to let other nurses know that they are doing a good job and that their hard work is recognized. They can promote a positive team environment in which they let the nurses know the importance of working together and making each other's lives better.

CULTURE OF RETENTION

A **culture of retention** is a place where people work that has values in place to keep them there. A culture of retention promotes employee satisfaction and preservation. Clinical nurse leaders can help to foster a culture of retention by recognizing the needs of the nursing staff and discovering how to best serve them. Within nursing, a culture of retention recognizes staff for their efforts and makes them feel valued. It considers the ideas of staff and attempts to implement them into practice. Nurse managers coach employees and make them feel valued for their hard work and competence. Nurses feel connected to one another and to management because they feel like they are working in a place where they matter. A culture of retention is more than bonuses and perks; it is an all-encompassing mindset that values all staff members who work together in the facility.

TYPES OF PEER-REVIEW PRACTICES

In the **peer-review process**, there are two major practices: incident-based peer review and safe-harbor peer review.

- **Incident-based peer review** occurs when an incident happens as a result of a nurse's work and the situation is reviewed to determine outcomes and discipline, if necessary. At times, major incidents that affect patients or staff may need to be peer-reviewed to evaluate the nurse's performance and determine what action is necessary, such as reporting to the state board of nursing.
- **Safe-harbor peer review** occurs when a nurse has concerns regarding her assigned practices. This type of review may happen if a nurse feels her work is beyond her scope of practice. The safe-harbor review process is designed to protect nurses from working beyond their licensing requirements as well as protect patients from receiving care from nurses who are not qualified to provide it.

PEER-REVIEW PROCESS COMPONENTS

- The **observation** component of the peer-review process involves gathering pertinent information about the activity of the nurse who is being reviewed. This may involve examining the nurse's professional duties or behavior. The nurse is notified of the observation process.
- **Feedback** occurs when the nurse is given information about performance, areas of strength, and areas of weakness. Feedback involves timely communication and direct honesty to allow the nurse to receive constructive criticism, which can help the nurse to make changes.
- The **strategizing** process addresses needs and concerns that are raised during peer review. If the nurse shows areas of weakness, strategizing works to develop a plan of improvement. Changes made must then be reinforced to promote continued positive development.

STEPS OF DESIGNING A PEER-REVIEW PROCESS

Steps of **designing a peer-review process**:

1. The initial step in developing a peer-review process is to get support for the process from the staff that will be participating. A planning group is then developed, which is focused on designing the peer-review process and educating staff about its methods. The group must decide how the process will be used among staff, such as through formal review or quality analysis.
2. The process of review is then designed, including components used to appraise the work of others, who will give feedback, and how results will be used.
3. Following design, nurses are educated about the peer-review process so they are aware of their roles. It is implemented for use among staff and after a period of time, evaluated for efficacy.
4. If there are issues determined during the evaluation process, the work group may then need to remedy those practices and revise the peer-review process to fit the needs of staff.

Communicating with the Patient

COMMUNICATION SKILLS

Effective communication by nurses is essential to provide adequate patient care and to meet patients' needs. Nurses can establish effective communication by asking questions of patients about what they expect from their care, from their stay in the hospital, or from their unit. Nurses also gather important information about their patients in case they have any needs to address regarding their care. Nurses must be good listeners to patients' concerns, questions, or comments about their care. Nurses must also put aside their own opinions or views that may affect the care of patients; additionally, they must let patients know that they are available to listen or discuss anything about which patients might need to talk.

CRITICAL-LISTENING SKILLS

Just as critical-thinking skills guide nurses for what action must be taken next in certain situations, **critical-listening skills** provide essential information that is gained only when nurses truly listen and attempt to understand their patients. Critical-listening skills may uncover data that could otherwise be missed in normal conversation but that are very important to the patients' care and well-being. Critical-listening skills involve not only hearing what patients are saying, but also recognizing body language and actions that may imply something else. Nurses do not interrupt or try to interject their own opinions or assumptions. Instead, they analyze what patients say, clarify the meaning if necessary, and determine if there are underlying feelings or thoughts that need to be explored.

VOICE MANAGEMENT

Voice management describes how nurses speak when they communicate with others. Among patients who have low health-literacy skills or language barriers, verbal communication is important to transmit important facts accurately about patients' situations. This is done by speaking clearly, avoiding the use of too many sentences, or avoiding the use of medical jargon. Voice management also describes how nurses speak, such as by using tone of voice and inflection. People who are native English speakers can often recognize when someone is using sarcasm or being condescending through their tone of voice. It is important for nurses to manage how they speak to avoid using tones that convey disrespect or irritation; even if nurses do not feel that way, these sentiments could inadvertently surface when they speak, so it is essential to practice voice control when speaking.

COMMUNICATING AS ADVANCED GENERALISTS

Because clinical nurse leaders act as advanced generalists, they are in a unique position to provide education and to increase communication with patients about their care, their current stay, and their priorities for treatment. Communication is an essential component of the role of advanced generalists. They must work as a translator for medical terms, by explaining potentially complicated medical concepts into a language that patients and families can understand. They may assist patients to participate in the work of the interdisciplinary team and educate them about their decisions about their own health. Advanced generalists listen carefully to patients and families to determine their point of view about care and the environment and then implement suggestions for change, when possible. Finally, advanced generalists consider the cultural needs of patients and determine how nursing care can still be effective if there are cultural differences, crossing barriers if any exist in the first place.

IMPROVING COMMUNICATION WITH PATIENTS

Health communication is an essential component of the job of clinical nurse leaders, and it is very important to ensure that there are no barriers to communication. Communication barriers may lead to misunderstandings about care, which can result in errors, complications, and increased costs. When providing information to patients, nurses can improve communication by speaking in a clear voice, rather than rambling or using a lot of medical jargon. They should use appropriate body language that conveys an open and friendly stance, which may make patients more comfortable asking questions. Nurses may use additional materials, such as pictures or media, to back up their teaching. If possible, nurses should ask patients to repeat the information back to them in their own words. Patients should be made to feel that asking questions is an appropriate response to teaching, rather than made to feel ashamed for asking.

POSITIVE THERAPEUTIC ALLIANCE

The **therapeutic alliance** between nurses and their patients promotes communication between caregivers and providers, supports the strengths of patients, and emphasizes how nurses can help patients. The therapeutic alliance involves nurses and patients working together for patient-focused care. This alliance affects the patients' mental and physical health. The relationship that develops between nurses and their patients may be warm and caring, helping patients to feel accepted and knowing that the nurses are working to meet their needs. Patients may develop an attitude of trust. Ideally, a positive therapeutic alliance may help patients to feel less anxious, insecure, depressed, or angry. Additionally, if patients are experiencing emotional stability because of the therapeutic alliance, they may have fewer physical symptoms and experience less severity of their disease. The therapeutic relationship recognizes the importance of both physical and mental health care to be a comprehensive care method for patients.

THERAPEUTIC COMMUNICATION

Therapeutic communication establishes an effective relationship between nurses and their patients and increases communication levels by reducing barriers. Nurses can practice therapeutic communication to get patients to disclose more information, feel more comfortable talking to them, or to reduce misunderstandings in the relationship. Some activities nurses can perform to increase therapeutic communication are addressing the patients by their preferred names, assessing patients' body language, listening without interrupting, respecting patients' cultural values and practices, and being honest with patients about their plan of care. Additionally, nurses should avoid disclosing too much personal information; they should allow patients to make as many choices as possible, and they should notify patients of changes in the treatment process.

SHARED DECISION-MAKING

Shared decision-making is the concept of working with patients to help them make the best decisions for their care and treatment. Shared decision-making allows patients to have a voice and participate in the plan of action for their care. Patients are given evidence-based information about treatments, management, screenings, and preferences. Shared decision-making is an important aspect of practice because it supports patients' viewpoints, giving them a feeling of empowerment over their own care. Because different people may respond to treatments or other practices in varied ways, there is no one method of making decisions. Instead, shared decision-making individualizes the care the patient receives. The process also supports the patients' cultural practices and beliefs if they do not otherwise agree.

POSITIVE REGARD

Positive regard is described as having respect for patients and seeing them as people of value and worth. Nurses must have positive regard for their patients to be able to care for them effectively and to provide care that meets their specific needs. Positive regard is more often conveyed through the behavior of nurses, rather than the words they use. Examples of actions that uphold positive regard for patients include paying attention to what patients are saying; using body language that conveys listening, such as a friendly posture, making eye contact, or nodding; remaining with patients during difficult times; and letting go of personal judgments or opinions that might affect patient care.

EMOTIONAL INTELLIGENCE

Salovey and Mayer developed the concept of **emotional intelligence** based on ability. Emotional intelligence is the ability to understand and manage one's own emotions as well as the ability to recognize and understand the emotions of others. Emotional intelligence is the understanding of how emotions affect behavior, a valuable skill in leaders. The four types of abilities involved in emotional intelligence include the ability to perceive, use, understand, and manage emotions. Individuals with emotional intelligence know the types of emotions that will be triggered personally by an event and have the ability to manage and use these emotions to enhance decision-making. They also can identify the emotions of others through observation of facial expressions, actions, words, and tone of voice. Individuals with emotional intelligence tend to have better social skills and workplace relationships because they have an innate understanding of how to respond to workers, to recognize their concerns, and to motivate them.

THERAPEUTIC RELATIONSHIP AND CONFLICT

The therapeutic relationship develops between the nurse and the patient as a consequence of daily communication about the patient's care. The therapeutic relationship is designed to be patient-centered: the nurse helps the patient with medical care and is a source of comfort and stability. **Conflict** can impede the therapeutic relationship if misunderstandings result in the development of mutual mistrust. A patient and nurse in conflict may be less likely to share important information about the patient's care. Conflict may cause hurt or angry feelings that can severely limit communication. It is important for the nurse to maintain appropriate lines of communication to ensure that conflict does not impede the therapeutic relationship and the nurse's role as someone who supports the patient.

RESPONSES TO CONFLICT

Conflict is inevitable in some health care situations, but with recognition of the appropriate **responses to conflict**, nurses can minimize conflict in the health care environment. Avoidance involves not actually dealing with the conflict. Instead, those who practice avoidance do not talk about it and pretend that conflict does not exist. This response causes everyone to lose because the conflict is not actually addressed. Accommodation involves allowing another person to have his way to resolve the conflict. This response may be appropriate in some situations, for instance, when continuing to disagree may cause more harm than good. Collaboration provides a win–win situation in that those in conflict can talk about the situation and work together to find a solution that works for everyone.

PROVIDING PRELIMINARY IMAGING RESULTS

Many patients who undergo radiologic exams want to know the results right away, particularly if they are facing a potentially significant disease. Patients often ask their nurses to tell them the results; however, without a radiologist present to conclude the findings, most technicians are not

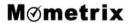

authorized to give this information. In some situations, patients are given their preliminary results before physicians sign their actual results, which could take several days or weeks. Preliminary results may give some patients peace of mind, leaving them with less worry while waiting for official results. Alternatively, many patients might want further information about their condition that nurses or technologists are unable to give. Ultimately, physicians must read the results and discuss them with their patients; while preliminary results may provide peace of mind for some, it can also backfire in situations in which the preliminary results are incorrect.

Written Communication

DEMONSTRATING ACCURATE NURSING DOCUMENTATION

Nursing documentation is an important component of nursing care, providing a record of the tasks that nurses have performed for patients and protecting them legally. There are several qualities that accurate nursing documentation should demonstrate. Nurses should fully describe the care given to their patients, including treatments, education, responses to treatment, and measures that demonstrate that they followed orders as prescribed. When nurses provide medication, they should document the type, dose, and time of administration and then document the patients' responses. Overall, nursing documentation should prove that the nurses provided care and should show that they took all steps necessary to provide reasonable and accurate care to the best of their ability.

DOCUMENTING INFORMED CONSENT

Informed consent is more than a piece of paper that a patient signs before a procedure. The process of obtaining informed consent involves a conversation between the patient and the physician, in which the physician explains the essential aspects of the procedure. Nurses must document that the patient was given this information and agreed to it, which is informed consent. Documentation of informed consent consists of evidence that the physician described the procedure, including its potential risks and complications, as well as the benefits and expected results of the procedure. Nurses must also document that their patients were told of the alternatives to the procedure, as well as their right to change to another health care provider if they decide to do so.

WRITTEN COMMUNICATION

Many people consider speaking and body language to be the essentials of communication, but **writing skills** are also important measures when educating patients or their families. Nurses must write regularly. Some nurses must write to educate patients about their conditions, their options for treatment, or their medication. In these cases, it is important to spell words correctly and to write clearly and legibly so that patients understand. The nurse should assess the patients' reading skills and vision before writing or presenting information that must be read to determine if they can understand it. If nurse is involved with writing educational materials, such as pamphlets or letters, they must use appropriate terminology that is easy to understand and free of errors. When information is not clear, patients may feel confused or may actually perceive the information incorrectly, reducing quality of care and possibly endangering their clinical situation.

Cultural Sensitivity

PROVIDING CULTURALLY COMPETENT PATIENT CARE

Nurses who recognize their patients' culture convey respect for the patients' belief system and cultural practices. Additionally, nurses who account for cultural differences understand that providing culturally sensitive care may result in an increased likelihood of patients listening to them and following through with treatment regimens. Nursing care that recognizes cultural differences may promote a positive relationship between patients and nurses. Patient may also have an easier time implementing ordered treatment measures when they comply with their cultural values and beliefs. Nurses who do not adhere to the recognized beliefs of patients when implementing teaching and care measures may be more likely to meet resistance from patients, which may develop into strained and unproductive relationships.

CULTURALLY COMPETENT HEALTH CARE SETTING

A **culturally competent health care setting** is one that recognizes that there are different sets of beliefs, values, and practices among patients and consumers, and it functions well with that knowledge. An environment that displays cultural competence shows respect for different cultures and takes steps to bridge gaps that may exist between patients, families, visitors, and staff. This may involve using language interpreters when language barriers are present. The organization may have signs in several languages to help patients avoid confusion about important health care information. The organization may need to provide instruction to health care providers so that they are aware of the different cultural practices they may encounter. Finally, the organization may attempt to hire clinicians with backgrounds similar to the patient populations.

SELF-REFLECTION

Before working with patients of different cultures, nurses must engage in **self-reflection** to assess their own beliefs and values. There may be times when nurses hold certain stereotypes regarding particular cultures, whether or not they are true. Nurses must assess what they know about the culture and consider any stumbling blocks that may prevent them from giving culturally sensitive care. Nurses must consider their own beliefs about themselves and their values; for instance, their beliefs about health and wellness, the role of health care organizations, their own religious or personal views, and their own views of such factors as gender or age. By engaging in self-reflection before providing care, nurses are able to examine and maintain their own beliefs so that they can give unbiased and sensitive care to their patients.

BUILDING RELATIONSHIPS IN THE COMMUNITY

Because many nurses regularly work with people from different cultural groups, it is important to take steps to understand better distinct differences, practices, beliefs, and feelings of those with different cultural backgrounds. Nurses should consider those groups about which they want to learn more by studying the culture through reading, attending religious or community events, or talking directly with members of the culture. They should strive to meet with as many people of the culture as possible to get a sense of their interests. Through the process of developing relationships with those from cultures different from nurses, they may better understand how to provide culturally relevant health care practices.

WORKING WITH LANGUAGE INTERPRETERS

Nurses who provide culturally sensitive care and who meet the cultural needs of patients may need to work with **language interpreters** to provide adequate education for some patients. When working with language interpreters, nurses should consider how the patient views the interpreter and remember that it is often a stranger who translates private medical information to the patient. Interpreters should be reminded to explain all of the information as the nurse presents it, rather than trying to use their own words, which can change the meaning. Nurses should still direct their discussions toward the patient and not the interpreter and avoid using complicated medical jargon while speaking. Before working with an interpreter, nurses must consider other factors that may affect the situation, such as the gender, age, and dialect of the interpreter.

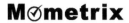

CULTURALLY RELEVANT HEALTH INFORMATION

Finding **culturally relevant health information** to provide effective and culturally sensitive care may be challenging for some nurses who lack time, resources, or understanding of how to begin. Nurses who want to find cultural information about a specific group may need to check the library, media, or the internet to first learn more about the group's practices, beliefs, and customs. If possible, nurses should try to attend a cultural event, particularly one that may incorporate health practices or beliefs to gain a better idea of a certain culture's expectations. Nurses could meet with both leaders and lay people from the group to talk about opportunities and ideas for care. Finally, some organizations that work with certain groups might offer presentations, seminars, or educational opportunities for learning more about specific practices for these groups.

ACCULTURATION

Acculturation is the process of one group or person taking on the cultural identities of another. Acculturation may occur in the health care setting if clinicians do not recognize the cultural practices that are important to certain patients. Patients with cultural practices that differ from those found in the hospital may try to hide their preferences or take on those of the health care team. Acculturation may work in an opposite way as well. Some nurses may decide to accept or participate in the cultural practices of their patients, even if they are very different from their former beliefs. This may be because they want to put their patients at ease or that they truly want to understand the beliefs and culture of their patients.

Quality Improvement Measures

QUALITY IMPROVEMENT

Quality improvement follows a process that carries ideas from beginning thoughts to implementation into care practice. For effective quality-improvement measures to take place, certain concepts must be in place.

- First, there must be **determination** toward commitment to quality improvement. Nurses and other staff must be willing to learn about the quality-improvement process, contribute ideas, and follow through with changes. Without determination, the quality-improvement cycle may quickly fold if everyone is not on board.
- **Ideas** consist of those thoughts or plans that contribute to quality improvement and that could be developed further through research or analysis.
- **Implementation** involves putting those ideas that have been proven to be effective for quality improvement into practice for the benefit of patients and staff.

RESEARCH AND PERFORMANCE-IMPROVEMENT MEASURES

Clinical research is performed to ask a question about a particular process or care standard. If a problem exists, clinical research can be done to attempt to solve the problem or to give insight into its management. Ultimately, research is performed so that the results can be applied within the clinical setting. In contrast, performance improvement is a process designed to develop better standards in practice.

Performance improvement might also be referred to as **quality improvement.** While research seeks to identify new information that can be applied to the clinical setting, performance improvement works to improve already existing care practices. Additionally, research results may be broadly distributed across various measures, while performance improvement is localized to the affected area.

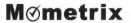

HOSPITAL QUALITY INITIATIVE

The **Hospital Quality Initiative** was started by the Centers for Medicare and Medicaid Services as a method of providing quality-improvement information to patients and consumers. Participation in the initiative is voluntary for health care organizations. It is designed to give information about quality practices of certain organizations so that consumers can make informed decisions about their care. It is also intended to support health care organizations as they seek to improve their quality-assessment measures. The public can access information about participating organizations and compare standards among organizations by going to the website at hospitalcompare.hhs.gov.

INTERDISCIPLINARY RESEARCH QUALITY INITIATIVE

The Robert Wood Johnson Foundation created the **Interdisciplinary Research Quality Initiative** in 2005 to determine how nurses impact quality of patient care and to use nurses as a source of improving standards that affect patient outcomes. Research outcomes have determined that high-quality care leads to better patient outcomes and less economic strain as a result of better compliance and a decreased risk of errors. The Quality Initiative provides information to managers, administrators, and policy makers about the importance of quality nursing care and its effects on patient outcomes, allowing them to make changes in policies, the environment, nursing practice guidelines, and laws that help drive high-quality care.

AGENCY FOR HEALTHCARE RESEARCH AND QUALITY

The **Agency for Healthcare Research and Quality (AHRQ)** is a branch of the US Department of Health and Human Services and receives funding from Congress. The AHRQ started in 1989 and seeks to promote quality health care measures, reduce costs, and encourage the use of evidence to guide practice and maintain competency in health care research. Much of the work of the AHRQ promotes evidence-based practice, and it has centers devoted to conducting research, the results of which can be implemented into clinical practice. The AHRQ also maintains a database of clinical practice guidelines. Called the National Guideline Clearinghouse, the website streamlines the process of finding guidelines for providers to use when they wish to improve practice standards.

MAGNET RECOGNITION PROGRAM MODEL

The **Magnet Recognition Program** is a recognition system for health care organizations that demonstrate quality, leadership, and excellence in nursing care. The Magnet Program Model from the American Nurses Credentialing Center guides those organizations that are seeking to apply for recognition from Magnet. The components of the program model include transformational leadership that guides organizations through their values and choices; structural empowerment, where staff practice professionally and have strong relationships; exemplary professional practice, which supports excellence in nursing care, autonomy, education, and interdisciplinary teamwork; improvements based on current research results; and structures for quality improvement.

NURSE RESIDENCY PROGRAM

Because of the increased demands nurses are facing in the clinical environment, more and more nurses are expected to perform clinical operations and critical thinking in highly stressful, challenging environments. Nurses are expected to make decisions that can affect practice, standards, and outcomes of care, even at very early points in their careers. Establishing a **nurse residency program** would provide a transitional period for nurses who have recently graduated to be supervised in their work in the clinical environment before being expected to do so on their own. This time of transition would be a learning experience beyond nursing school that provides individualized instruction for the specific area where the new nurse is employed. A nurse residency program ultimately affects patient outcomes because new nurses who are assigned to patients will

91

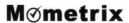

have more background and education in the particular area, enabling them to make decisions and to practice accurately because they have received extra training to transition into their roles as nurses.

QUALITY-IMPROVEMENT INITIATIVES

When deciding to implement **new measures of quality improvement**, nurses must often compare these ideas with other models to measure standards. Measures used for comparisons are often already being used in current practice and have proven to be effective. These measures should also be related to the new ideas for implementation; they should be specific and allow the nurse doing the comparison to be able to evaluate the results. The measures should also be applicable to the current situation or unit of practice. For instance, if nurses are comparing new ideas for quality improvement in reducing the incidence of catheter-associated urinary infections, they should compare the new ideas with current measures of practice that reveal outcomes appropriate for populations who use catheters and who are, therefore, at greatest risk for these infections.

FOSTERING QUALITY IMPROVEMENT WITHIN MICROSYSTEMS

The **culture of the microsystem** has an impact on quality improvement, and several **strategies** may be implemented that can foster improved methods of providing quality care. Some examples of strategies include expectations of staff that are clear and communicated well about supporting quality-improvement measures, developing a cultural belief that quality is the responsibility of all staff, maintaining accountability for quality among all staff members, developing quality councils comprised of nurses and physicians who research quality-improvement practices, and providing feedback to nursing staff regarding their efforts at improving quality care.

IMPROVING WORKFLOW

In clinical nursing, **workflow** might entail providing patient care, determining lab results, calling physicians, and talking with family members. When workflow runs smoothly, tasks are completed in a timely manner. When interruptions disrupt the workflow, frustration can result. Clinical nurse leaders can improve workflow among nurses by assessing whether implemented strategies are truly helping. For example, one of the benefits of electronic health records (EHRs) is to streamline documentation, but if nurses must continually manage technical glitches to use EHRs, their workflow is interrupted. Clinical nurse leaders must look for ways to help nurses increase productivity without disruptions in care by assessing policies to determine the length of time to implement practices, checking standards to clarify if they are time-consuming, or considering nurse–patient ratios to ensure that work burdens are not too heavy.

SUPPORTING QUALITY CARE

High-quality patient care is a goal of most organizations that wish to break down barriers that prevent patients from receiving such care. Many organizations have **vision statements** or **goals** centered on providing high-quality care, and they continuously try to implement strategies that will support this care. Organizations may take on a **patient-focused mindset**, in which patients' needs are always considered, including the needs of new medical practices, sensitive and focused care, excellence in nursing staff, and capabilities for complaints or evaluations. An organization may also **recognize staff members** who provide outstanding care by rewarding them so they will continue to practice high-quality medicine. Other strategies include consulting evidence-based practice to uphold care standards, promoting quality and safety initiatives, and reaching out to various patient populations to ensure that their needs are met in the community.

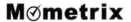

HAND HYGIENE

Hand hygiene is one of the most common and easily applied forms of infection control in the clinical environment. Education about and access to appropriate hand hygiene materials can improve compliance and ultimately reduce the incidence of infection. Nurses may work to implement several types of interventions to improve hand hygiene among colleagues, staff, patients, and visitors. Posting signs of the benefits of hand washing and its reduction in disease near sinks reminds people of the importance of hand washing. Some clinical care environments have waterless hand sanitizers available at nursing stations and within patients' rooms for easy access. Sinks within rooms should be automatic so that nurses can avoid turning water on and off by hand and spreading germs in the process. Nurses should take measures to wash their hands carefully, follow policies regarding jewelry, and sanitize equipment after use to reduce the spread of potentially infectious organisms among patients.

STRUCTURAL DESIGN

Interventions and evidence-based practices are not the only activities that affect patient outcomes. The **structure** of a health care facility can impact patients' overall health and potential for adverse outcomes. Depending on how a facility is designed, patients may be less likely to acquire hospital-based infections; less likely to have adverse events, such as falls; and may improve at a faster pace due to patients' satisfaction with their care. For example, the incidence of hospital-acquired infections may be better managed through environmental changes, such as having adequate ventilation systems or access to enough sinks for hand washing. Patients may be less likely to fall if their environment does not contain structures that act as obstacles when ambulating. Rooms that are pleasant, temperature-controlled, and quiet may contribute to patient satisfaction, potentially increasing quality of care and possibly better outcomes.

INDOOR AIR QUALITY

Indoor air quality has the potential to impact patient outcomes significantly because it describes the quality of circulating air throughout the facility. If the air is low quality, patients and staff may suffer. Poor indoor air quality may contribute to hospital-based infections if pathogens are allowed to travel through the air or ventilation systems and infect other patients or staff members. The health care center must have an adequate HVAC system in place to prevent the transmission of infection through the air. Some facilities must have negative-pressure rooms that circulate so that patients with airborne infectious diseases have less chance of infecting others. Air quality also impacts comfort levels of patients and staff, and patients may have more positive psychological outcomes with good air quality. Nurses are also more likely to consider their environment positively if good air quality is maintained, allowing them to give more effective care to patients.

ACTIVITIES TO INCREASE THE SATISFACTION OF PATIENTS

The outpatient setting offers access to care in the community, but patients who are seeking services may have a choice as to where they want to have their services provided. Nurses can increase the **satisfaction of patients** at their location, which may bring patients back on repeated visits when they need further care, rather than finding a different provider. Nurses should show flexibility with scheduling, if at all possible, by meeting patients where they are and at the specific hours that work best. Serving as liaisons is another method by which nurses work to increase communication between patients and physicians. Nurses can also ensure that patients have adequate information about clinic hours, where to pick up prescriptions, and when to return. If there are patients with low health-literacy skills or who have trouble understanding forms, nurses can help fill out paperwork or teach the patients how to do it themselves.

QUALITY IMPROVEMENT DRAWBACKS

While new initiatives are being offered on a regular basis as methods of evaluating quality, too many initiatives increase pressure on staff to perform up to the highest standards. There is nothing wrong with desiring high-quality standards; in fact, hospitals should make high-quality standards part of their goals. However, with new initiatives being introduced frequently, it may be difficult for organizations to keep up with changes. Hospitals may find that some practices, while evidence-based, duplicate what they already perform. They may have adequate standards in place, but with new initiatives, their policies may need to be revised on a frequent basis to stay current. Finally, many nurses are already overworked from providing bedside care; thus, they do not have much time to devote to revising quality standards constantly. Health care centers may need to consider each new initiative as it comes to determine whether its implementation will be beneficial to the facility and staff.

Safety

SAFETY OF PATIENTS

Because the **safety of patients** is of utmost importance for most health care organizations, there may be similar attributes between organizations that promote safety. Organizations that recognize the importance of quality assurance and the provision of high-quality care, as well as those that are willing to implement changes in practice guidelines to reflect greater safety goals often openly promote the safety of patients. Additionally, organizations that maintain employee morale promote the safety of patients, as nurses who feel good about their jobs may be less likely to make errors in clinical care. Other examples include organizations that consider nurse-to-patient ratios for care, those that recognize work demands among nurses, those that promote professional growth and provide educational assistance for staff, and those that offer supportive leadership are all classified as promoting greater levels of safety for their patients.

ERRORS OF OMISSION AND ERRORS OF COMMISSION

Patient safety involves improving quality of care to reduce negative outcomes and to protect patients from harm. While nurses often make the safety of patients a high priority of their care, errors still occur.

- **Errors of omission** are those that happen when nurses fail to provide a service for which they were responsible, such as when medication aides fail to provide a medication, physical therapists do not administer prescribed therapy as ordered, or nurses do not arrange for further services as ordered by the physician.
- **Errors of commission** include times when nurses perform an incorrect act. Examples include if medication aides provide medication but in the wrong dose or if physical therapists perform the wrong therapy for the patient's condition.

BARCODE MEDICATION ADMINISTRATION

Scanning a patient's barcode, which is typically found on a wristband, before administering medication is a benefit of **barcode medication administration.** The associated computer has the information about the medication available, including the dose and the timing of its administration. The system is designed to reduce errors in medication administration by providing another check for safety before giving medicine. Barcode administration may reduce errors in medication administration by reducing instances of wrong patients, wrong dosages, or wrong timing of medications. Alternatively, not all patients can wear the barcode on their person; for example, infants. Barcodes could be inadvertently mixed up or unavailable, which may result in incorrect

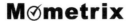

dosages given. Additionally, nurses must still answer the rights of medication administration before giving medication and not totally rely on the barcode system to prevent errors.

Nurse Staffing Issues

Nurse staffing issues may greatly impact the safety of patients, sometimes negatively, including an increased number of sentinel events and increased levels of morbidity and mortality. When nursing units are short staffed, the nurse-to-patient ratio may be lower than safely recommended. This increases the risk for errors that can jeopardize the safety of patients. Additionally, the level of training of staff nurses may also affect the safety of nurses. Nurses may have different levels of education, and many nursing units offer only a short time of training to learn the many dynamics of the unit. This can also result in more frequent errors as less-educated nurses or those who have not been trained adequately within specific care settings may be providing ineffective care, resulting in more mistakes. Those who manage staffing issues need to account for various skill mixes and ratios of nurses to patients, which are complex processes that require practice to protect the safety of all patients.

Safety Concepts

Clinical nurse leaders act as resources for educating and supporting others in seeking and maintaining the safety of patients. Clinical nurse leaders must recognize when constraints exist that may affect the unit's ability to provide safe and effective care. If there are safety issues, clinical nurse leaders notify the right personnel who can address and correct these issues. Additionally, clinical nurse leaders ensure that financial resources are allocated to provide education to staff about upholding the safety of patients. If necessary, these leaders must ensure that policies reflect the safety goals of the organization. Finally, clinical nurse leaders are responsible for evaluating if changes made to promote safe practices are viable, if these changes support the safety goals of the organization, or if they need to be amended.

Waste Management

Most organizations separate the **waste products** from central areas of functioning. While hospitals and health care centers often do this as well, there are times when high-risk materials may need to be near areas where care is provided. Nurses promote safety in the environment by carefully containing waste products or toxins so that they do not cause harm to patients or visitors. This may involve storing items properly so that they are out of sight and out of reach of the public, disposing of certain toxic or sharp materials in the appropriate receptacles, and labeling receptacles with specific details about their contents. Additionally, the nursing unit should have safety data sheets with information about each type of material used, the effects of its exposure, and what to do in case of contact.

Vigilance

In nursing, **vigilance** is described as paying attention to the environment, closely watching situations to determine when change is occurring, assessing risk in caring for patients, and responding appropriately to changes in patients' conditions. Vigilance affects patient outcomes in that the behavior of nurses may track changes that can significantly affect patients' conditions. For example, when nurses are vigilant about patient care, they may notice subtle changes that point to deterioration. They can then notify providers for further orders to correct the situation, ultimately impacting outcomes. Thus, vigilance is a component of caring that is the essence of nursing care that impacts patient outcomes through interventions.

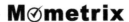

FINANCIAL EFFECTS OF PATIENTS' INJURIES

The financial effects of patients' injuries are enormous for health care organizations that must provide care for patients who have been injured in their facilities and often must absorb some of the costs of providing that care. Patients who receive Medicaid or Medicare services and who become injured while in the hospital will not be covered by the Centers for Medicare and Medicaid Services. In other words, if a patient whose health care is normally covered through Medicare becomes injured or develops an illness while in the hospital, Medicare will not pay for the added care it requires to treat that patient. This increases the importance of regular risk assessments in the clinical environment to reduce instances of injuries and illnesses, such as patient falls or infections.

SENTINEL EVENT

A **sentinel event** is defined by the Joint Commission as an event that is unintended, and causes death or significant physical or psychological injury or the risk of this occurring. A sentinel event is so significant that it requires investigation following its occurrence, and health care organizations must have systems in place that actively seek to reduce or eliminate sentinel events in their facilities. Some reasons why sentinel events occur include poor communication, incorrect assessment of patients' conditions, failure to report changes in patients' conditions, poor training on the part of health care providers, poor coordination among providers during transitional periods, inaccurate handoffs of patients, over-dependence on medical technology that resulted in malfunction, and shortages in nursing staff.

INCIDENT REPORT

An **incident report** is a document that should be filled out after an adverse incident occurs that affects a patient, family, or staff. An incident report is filed to allow risk managers to assess what circumstances are causing risk for those in the health care environment and to determine where changes should be made in practice. Many reports are form templates that involve filling in blanks. Nurses should be sure to record the date and time of the incident, the people involved, and facts about what happened. They should ensure that they give only the facts and refrain from giving opinions. This involves avoiding blame for what happened. The incident report should be filled out as quickly as possible after the event, while the information is still fresh in the nurses' minds. Each organization has their own policy for reporting incident reports; nurses should know to whom to forward the documents and should follow the chain of command for filing them.

NEAR MISS ERROR

A **near miss** is a situation that had the potential to cause harm, increase illness, or result in death, but actually did not do so. When a near miss occurs, nurses should consider the circumstances surrounding the event and what changes can be made to prevent the event from actually occurring. For example, if nurses realize that they are preparing to give patients an unsafe dose of medication and then stop themselves, they are experiencing a near miss. Nurses can analyze these situations to determine where they made the mistake—such as by failing to check the medication with another person or failing to check the order—and then incorporate a change in practice to prevent this from happening again. Near misses can result in better patient outcomes because practice changes can ultimately protect the safety of patients.

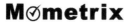

Data Analysis

PATIENT REGISTRY

A **patient registry** is a system that collects data about patient outcomes related to specific groups of people. For example, a certain patient registry may consist of information about patient outcomes related to patients with ovarian cancer while another registry may have outcome data related to patients with chronic obstructive pulmonary disease. The registry may take information from research studies or other methods of collection to gather data. A patient registry may be created to guide caregivers in their interventions with specific diseases, to discern cost-effectiveness of certain practices related to specific diseases, to measure quality standards in patient care, or to maintain the safety of patients when providing care.

ASSESSING PRODUCT SAFETY

Product registries may assist nurses in the evaluation of the safety and quality of patient care through the use of certain items, administration of certain medications, or the use of certain therapeutic interventions. Product registries have been developed in response to previous negative side effects that have occurred after implementation of certain activities in the past. They are now used to evaluate the safety and effectiveness of certain medications, therapies, or interventions to provide surveillance for potential adverse outcomes that could occur. Clinicians who use product registries are willing to understand the limitations of their interventions as well as acknowledge potentially negative effects.

COLLECTION METHODS OF QUALITATIVE DATA

Qualitative research identifies factors that are difficult to measure in actual numbers, such as behavior, motivation, assumptions, or goals. **Qualitative data collection** often requires contact with participants to determine their background through discussion or observation to gain valuable data for research. Examples of methods in which nurses may collect data for qualitative analysis include participant interviews, focus groups, direct observations, background and ethnographic review, medical or life history, questionnaires or surveys, medical records and documentation, or videotaping. Some methods of collection may be intrusive toward participants, such as interviews, while other methods may affect participants very little, such as reviewing medical records or performing cultural reviews.

METHODS USED FOR SAMPLING QUALITATIVE DATA

Qualitative data sampling may consist of one of three methods.

- **Purposive sampling**, the most common, seeks to select samples according to the particular research question or the number of participants available who are appropriate for the specific data needed.
- **Snowball sampling** uses the contacts of those participants already involved to gain new participants for the study. Snowball sampling may use resources, such as social networks, to connect people in common who may all be candidates for the study and to get them involved as active participants.
- In **quota sampling**, the researcher determines how many participants are needed for the study and what particular characteristics they must have to be involved. This type of sampling helps the researchers to narrow the possibilities for participants to those which they believe would provide the most appropriate outcomes.

DESCRIPTIVE STATISTICS AND INFERENTIAL STATISTICS

Quantitative research is performed with data that can be calculated and are measurable. The results in quantitative research are often presented statistically, which may take several forms.

- **Descriptive statistics** are those that provide a summary of the results of a study. Descriptive statistics use such measures as central tendency (median, mean, or mode) or measures of variability (standard deviation) to describe outcomes of the research data that were measured.
- **Inferential statistics** are processes that must be calculated to help the researcher understand or predict what the process might be. Examples of inferential statistics include calculating the probability of a certain event occurring or finding the statistical significance of an event.

NURSING SURVEILLANCE

Surveillance is the process of acquiring patient data, interpreting results, and analyzing the information to determine what actions are appropriate and where changes must be made. Surveillance is essential for providing appropriate patient care and preventing adverse outcomes. While patient monitoring is part of surveillance, there is more to surveillance than just monitoring. Patient monitoring should take up a large component of surveillance in that nurses receive information about patients through monitoring and analyze it for changes or effects. Surveillance then continues beyond monitoring to impact nursing interventions, identify errors, and discover areas that cause complications.

CLINICAL QUALITY VALUE ANALYSIS

A **Clinical Quality Value Analysis** may be performed at the time of decision-making for new products or services within an organization. This type of analysis helps decision-makers to recognize whether certain products or services are valuable to their organization, financially stable, and will improve patient outcomes. The value analysis involves assessing the products and their specifications. Next, the analysis determines the plan for the product, such as how or when it would be used and where it should be implemented. The design of the product and the design of the organization are taken into consideration as well as the impact of using the product. If the measures point toward a positive recommendation for using the product, it is then implemented into practice. Finally, following implementation, the analysis requires evaluation of the success of the product and how well it upholds quality and integrity, according to the organization's guidelines.

GAP ANALYSIS

Gap analysis considers a company's current performance with what it could be. Within health care, gap analysis takes into account an organization's actual activities, such as staffing patterns, patterns of spending, fiscal responsibility, and care standards, and compares those factors with what they could be. This comparison is designed to not only recognize the current performance of the institution but to set a goal for where it should be within a certain time frame. Gap analysis recognizes the investments of organizations into their time and resources. It acts as a form of benchmarking against itself to continue to improve its own measures and capabilities for performance.

USING GAP ANALYSIS TO DEVELOP AN EFFECTIVE HEALTH CARE TEAM

Nurses use gap analysis to consider those practices and resources they currently have available as compared to what they want to be doing. When **developing an effective health care team**, nurses should consider the team currently working in their environment: their strengths, weaknesses, and overall effectiveness. They should then consider what they want out of a team, such as success in

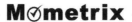

making changes to the environment, maintaining accountability, and supporting patient-focused care. After determining what they have and what they want, nurse leaders look at the measures before them to determine what should be upheld and what should be changed. They consider measures that they can implement to meet the goals of the team. Finally, they plan for future use of gap analysis to maintain evaluation of current and prospective work of care teams.

ROOT-CAUSE ANALYSIS ACTION PLAN

When a sentinel event occurs in a health care organization, those involved must determine whether the event was significant enough that it requires reporting to higher-level organizations, such as the state health department or the Joint Commission. A **root-cause analysis** is performed to determine what factors were associated with the event occurring and what activities led up to the sentinel event. This analysis must be performed within 45 days of the event so that the details are still fresh. If the event is reported, the organization devises an analysis action plan that describes the event and the organization's efforts to prevent it from recurring. The action plan should explain the changes made by the organization, the timeline for the changes, how the new methods are monitored, and how new methods and standards are evaluated for effectiveness. These descriptions are all put into the action plan to describe the organization's action for the prevention of future sentinel events.

SECONDARY ANALYSIS

Nurses who use evidence-based practice to guide their care standards may implement these practices, according to policy or facility requirements. There may be times when further questions are needed based on evidence-based practice results, such as when the data must be updated or if there is a specific situation that is not necessarily covered under the practice results and requires further study. A **secondary analysis** may be indicated in these situations. A secondary analysis is performed by questioning completed data and reviewing it again to obtain answers. This process may be performed on different types of practice results, such as formal nursing research results or other data collection measures. For example, if nurses questioned a certain infection-control practice at their workplace that was implemented because of evidence-based results, they may choose to perform a secondary analysis to clarify which procedures are appropriate for the infection-control practices and if they specifically apply to their current situation.

RISK ANALYSIS

Increased patient acuity, increased use of technology and staffing shortages are just some of the reasons why **risk analysis** is important in clinical nursing. Patient safety is often at risk because of the number of treatments and therapies that may be necessary, as well as the clinical environment itself. This safety risk must be continuously assessed and analyzed to make changes in practice that will keep patients safe. The role of risk analysis is to prevent accidents or injuries from occurring and to make the health care center a safe and quality place for patients. Risk analysis is also essential to protect nursing staff. By monitoring how nurses perform their work, risk analysis protects staff against physical, emotional, or legal actions.

QUANTITATIVE AND QUALITATIVE RISK ANALYSIS

Nurses may use two **types of risk analysis** to examine factors that put their patients at risk.

- **Quantitative analysis of risk** uses statistical results to explain risk in an environment. Quantitative results are measurable and include hard facts that can be calculated. For example, nurses might use quantitative analysis of the number of bed sores that have developed in the last year on their unit by performing research related to associated variables in this situation.

- **Qualitative analysis of risk** is more descriptive and asks questions, such as what could happen in this situation, or what is the outcome if this negative event occurs? Using the bed-sore example, nurses might analyze how bedsores occur and examine patient-care measures to determine how likely is it that bedsores will occur in certain groups.

INTRINSIC AND EXTRINSIC RISK FACTORS

Risk assessments in the patient environment must include both intrinsic factors and extrinsic factors.

- **Intrinsic factors** are those factors that are related to patients and their health. For example, patients at risk for falls may have difficulties with walking or cognitive changes; patients at risk for infection may have a lowered immune system because of medications.
- **Extrinsic factors** are those items in the environment that may contribute harm to patients and put them at risk of adverse outcomes. Patients at risk for falling may have extrinsic risk factors, such as clutter in the room or a wet floor. Patients may be at increased risk for infection due to extrinsic factors, such as failure of the nursing staff to perform adequate hand hygiene.

METHODS OF COLLECTING DATA

When determining risk factors in the clinical environment, nurses must use not only their clinical judgment but also several methods for collecting information that can be applied to risk analysis.

- **Observations** are those situations in which nurses monitor activity, watch situations around them, and use their senses or a gut instinct to gather data about patients' risks.
- **Interviewing** allows nurses to determine risk by talking with patients and taking their medical histories, especially about their current situations. Nurses may gain a lot of information through interviewing that can lead their interventions toward increased safety.
- The **physical examination** also gives nurses physical cues about patients' conditions, which allows them to assess risk, such as through patients' levels of mobility, presence of infection, or concurrent diagnoses that may lead to increased risk.

CLINICAL NURSING EXPERIENCE

Past experience of nurses may help them to understand current risk factors that prevent patient safety. If, for example, nurses witness or experience episodes that result in negative outcomes for patients, they may be more likely to remember these episodes when they experience something similar. For example, if nurses have had patients fall while caring for then, they may remember the risk factors associated with those falls and assess for them with their future patients.

Additionally, **instincts** of nurses may be based not only on what they have learned in training but also on their "gut feeling" that something is not entirely right. This instinct may allow nurses to reassess the current situation and determine the presence of risk factors.

RISK ANALYSIS FOR PATIENT FALLS

Assessing for patient safety is the role of all nurses, and those who care for **patients at risk for falls** must be aware of factors that increase the risk. When assessing for fall risk, nurses must consider the patients' ages and if they have fallen before; if they use assistive devices, such as walkers or canes; if they have a medical background that may affect their mobility, such as obesity, arthritis, history of hip or knee surgery, or diabetes; and if patients have visual disturbances. Additionally, nurses should assess the cognitive status of patients and their use of medications that may affect balance or vision. The physical environment should be assessed for risk of causing falls,

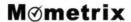

such as wet floors or objects in the way. Additionally, nurses who assess fall risks for patients must consider what patients wear and if these clothes increase their risk of falling, such as long clothing or socks.

RISK MANAGEMENT NURSE

Clinical nurse leaders who are also **risk managers** contribute to the safety of both patients and staff. As risk managers, nurses look for areas of liability to the health care organization or areas that could potentially cause harm to patients, families, nurses, or other staff. Types of liabilities may be physical, emotional, or financial. Nurses must take into consideration any legal claims that patients have taken against the organization, respond to patient complaints, consider financial statements to look for signs of fraud or abuse, review the work of staff nurses to ensure they are not engaging in activities that could be a liability to the organization, and educate others about the importance of risk management. Risk-management nurses must have a background in medical treatments, legal proceedings, and fiscal management and must be aware of laws and regulations that affect health care systems.

RISK MANAGERS

One of the roles of clinical nurse leaders is as **risk managers** for those with whom they work. Clinical nurse leaders must assess risk among both their patients and their colleagues. They determine which patients are at risk because of safety concerns associated with the unit or discrepancies in quality care. They may participate in research to determine which unit factors contribute to patient illness or infection and make changes based on outcome. They may also assess risk among their colleagues to determine who is participating in health and wellness activities, as mismanagement of health among nursing staff contributes to decreased productivity and lost work time. Clinical nurse leaders may also act as nurses in the chain of command when staff nurses need assistance with their tasks or guidance as to how to handle situations that are not clear to minimize the risk of adverse outcomes.

QUALITY-IMPROVEMENT MEASURES

On some clinical units, teams of nurses or clinicians are developed to analyze quality-improvement measures and determine what methods are currently working and what should be revised. Quality-improvement teams may meet to discuss ideas. The team may be able to visit other sites and use the information as a benchmark for their own ideas about what quality-improvement methods work in the clinical environment. All members of the team may have their own projects or tasks to be completed between meetings, and group meetings call for updates in practice on the projects currently underway. Ultimately, the team is called to discuss quality-improvement measures, implement them into clinical practice, educate others about the importance of quality improvement, and train others to develop new ideas for quality improvement.

Evidence-Based Practice

Evidence-based practice uses research outcomes to drive the best methods of nursing care. Nurses can use evidence-based practice throughout their careers. They may use research outcomes to apply specific practices where they work, or they may change their policies based on these practices. Reading the results of research provides current information that may differ from what nurses learned in training. Evidence-based practice keeps nurses current throughout their careers instead of using outdated practice methods. Nurses may also use evidence-based practice as part of lifelong learning if they participate in research studies that examine new practice methods. Performing research is informative, and determining the outcomes teaches research nurses new information about the research process.

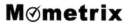

EVIDENCE-BASED PRACTICE AND RESEARCH

Evidence-based practice considers a question or task and looks at evidence available that either supports or opposes the topic to guide practice. Nurses may use research for evidence-based practice to search information, but they may also use other sources, such as expert opinion, quality-improvement data, or information gained during training.

Alternatively, **research** is the process of creating new knowledge about a topic or answering a question about a specific subject. Research then uses a specific process to gather information, analyze the data, and report the results. Research results are often used to support evidence-based practice but are not the same concept.

NURSING RESEARCH

Nursing research is an important part of disseminating evidence-based practice information to other nurses so they can implement it into their own standards of care. Quality nursing research always discusses the problem or issue at hand or asks a question about some aspect of nursing practice. The research information provided should be accurate and based on methods performed to reach outcomes. The research that is done follows standards for ethical practice in how participants are involved. The research may be repeatable, in that other nurses could potentially replicate the study and publish their results. The written report discusses any shortcomings of the research method and how they affected the process. Finally, research is often published, following a specific method of describing the activities, outcomes, and discussion of the project.

RESEARCH PROCESS STEPS

Nursing research follows a process that is designed to introduce the information and follow through the steps of the activity until a conclusion is reached. Clinical nurse leaders initially formulate questions that can be answered by research, such as information regarding clinical practice activities. They then review any literature or studies that may already be related to the issue. Clinical nurse leaders develop a hypothesis for the study and then determine what type of study design is most applicable. If research participants are needed, they are separated into groups, if applicable. Nurse leaders then conduct the study and collect needed data to analyze the results. After all data are collected, the nurses review and analyze outcomes. They then write about or discuss their findings, which may later be published or otherwise disseminated for review.

TYPES OF OBSERVATIONAL STUDIES

Observational studies are a certain type of research study that nurses may encounter in practice and literature review. These studies do not change the variables involved, rather they observe and record how outcomes progress.

- **Panel studies** are those in which a group is observed over a period of time. In panel studies, the original sets of participants are used throughout the study, with no variation in population.
- **Cohort studies** also observe a group of people over time; however, members of the group may change if observations are repeated.
- **Case-control studies** compare groups of people who are classified into different groups; for instance, a case-control study may observe the behaviors of patients diagnosed with mental illness and patients who do not have mental health diagnoses.

META-ANALYSIS

Meta-analysis is a type of study in which nurses look at research results from various studies and analyze the results. This is a quantitative process, and rather than performing new research and gathering participants, nurses use information from studies that have been completed. Nurses may gather research outcomes from several studies that are focused on the same topic. They then identify the results from the different studies and review them to make comparisons. The data are then statistically analyzed, and results may be applied to nursing standards. The meta-analysis provides a comprehensive review of research outcomes from various sources about a particular topic. This method can increase certainty in particular practices or processes because it has the backing of research results from several different studies.

SYSTEMATIC REVIEW

A **systematic review** is a literature review to search for evidence to be used to support or change practice standards. A systematic review is a comprehensive approach to locating literature sources, evaluating their appropriateness for inclusion, and synthesizing relevant information. The nurse uses a search database to perform a wide search of literature and then systematically assesses the results. Those potential sources are narrowed down to examples of the highest quality and most appropriate for the situation. Nurses can perform a systematic review when they want to find evidence to back up their practices or to find sources of new information that can eventually be applied to patient-care practices.

BARRIERS TO PERFORMING A SYSTEMATIC REVIEW

Although there are many different sources available for searching literature to be applied toward evidence-based practices, nurses may encounter **barriers** that prevent them from completing a review. There are some databases used for searching, which can be found in medical libraries or online and can narrow down searches to specific topics. However, nurses may have difficulty navigating the system or may not understand how to use it. They may search using terms that are too broad, which provides too many results and slows the process of sifting through available literature. Some literature may come up in a search that is unpublished and, therefore, inaccessible; additionally, nurses may have difficulty locating actual copies of the sources listed in results. In some cases, copies of sources must be accessed through interlibrary loan or transport of materials to another location.

NURSING PRACTICE RESEARCH COUNCIL

Some units use clinical nurse leaders and staff nurses to research evidence-based practices that are specific to their patient populations and the results can be implemented into unit standards. Forming a **nursing practice research council** benefits nurses and their patients in several ways. The nurses who serve on the council become familiar with the research process and learn to identify best practices through evidence-based results. The group may consist of staff from several levels, including staff nurses, clinical nurse leaders, and administrators. This variety of in-group members may improve communication and relationships among those who must work together. The group consults certain research designs and determines which methods can be implemented into practice. The group may also be responsible for educating staff about these new methods, as well as evaluating their effectiveness. Patients benefit from these practice councils because they receive care from nurses with experience in the dissemination of research outcomes. They also receive up-to-date care that is based on evidence-based practices.

NURSING RESEARCH ARTICLE

Many **nursing research articles** follow a format that consists of several components that follow a certain progression; each stage covers essential material of the study that makes the information easy to identify and locate within the article. The title provides a very brief explanation of the topic or question being researched; studies also publish the author's name and credentials below the title. The abstract consists of a synopsis of the information presented in the article, including the results. The introduction is the next section, and this segment presents the information and reasons for performing the research. The methods section describes how the research was carried out, how the study was designed, and how the participants were selected. The results section explains the findings from the research. The discussion section is often the final section, which reviews the findings and results, discusses their reliability, and considers questions raised throughout the process.

KNOWLEDGE TRANSFER OF EVIDENCE-BASED PRACTICES

The Agency for Healthcare Research and Quality model of evidence-based practice identifies three phases of **knowledge transfer** when developing and using evidence-based practices.

1. The first stage, **knowledge creation and distillation**, involves performing research and then providing recommendations for clinical practice based on the results.
2. The second step is **diffusion and dissemination**, which distributes the information to users. The researchers may need to partner with other organizations to disseminate information, such as through journal articles or professional nursing organizations.
3. Finally, end-user adoption, **implementation**, and institutionalization occur when health care systems adopt the practices supported by evidence-based practice, which is based on research findings. This may involve changing current policies and evaluating outcomes based on findings until the new methods of performance are fully integrated into clinical practice.

TRANSLATION SCIENCE

Translation science considers the factors that affect adoption and implementation of evidence-based practice that may be used to improve clinical standards of care. Translation science is concerned with factors that may be preventing the implementation of evidence-based practices and looks for ways to overcome barriers. The process may include promoting outcomes of studies designed to improve care, considering the attitudes of staff toward evidence-based practices, or analyzing past implementation of new information. Once armed with this information, the process of translation science can then educate those using evidence-based methods about their importance. Following implementation, translation science may be necessary to evaluate how well participants are using evidence-based practices as well as what processes must be changed.

LOCATING EVIDENCE THAT SUPPORTS EVIDENCE-BASED PROTOCOLS

Locating evidence is an early step in developing evidence-based practice that will eventually support or change current protocols and standards of clinical care. Nurses must first determine the subject area for which they want to search, such as protocols regarding the risk of falls or best practices for wound management. Based on the topic, nurses can then use literature reviews to find evidence, such as nursing journals, textbooks, or review articles. The nurse should understand research concepts and how to analyze research results. Use of certain database tools, such as the *Cumulative Index to Nursing and Allied Health Literature*, may also be necessary to foster better search results. If possible, a librarian at the hospital library who specializes in health care research may be able to help to find sources for a literature review. Once the appropriate amount of evidence is found to support or oppose their claims, nurses may then take steps toward change.

CUMULATIVE INDEX OF NURSING AND ALLIED HEALTH LITERATURE

The *Cumulative Index of Nursing and Allied Health Literature* **(CINAHL)** is a database that can be searched for various articles and publications that may be used in practice and is typically available in medical libraries or online. Nurses can access CINAHL to find information from journals, books, dissertations, conference materials, and educational offerings. Accessing CINAHL helps nurses in their search for literature as part of the review process for evidence-based practice. It may also be used for finding information to support data for writing or presenting, or finding sources of data for class work. Nurses who do not understand how to access CINAHL may learn relatively quickly from a medical librarian. The database has searchable measures that can narrow down fields to specific topics or sources that can help nurses to identify the most appropriate information for their purposes.

INFORMATION LITERACY

Information literacy consists of the knowledge of and ability to determine when information needs to be sought, how to research and locate pertinent information, and how to consider its results for practice. Nurses must be information literate to maintain their current skills and knowledge, as well as to remain updated about new practices that should be implemented into care. Information literacy is required for literature searches when researching results of evidence-based practice; it may also be necessary in such situations as knowing how or where to find information that can be given to patients about their current conditions. Nurses need to be information literate if they take educational courses to continue their education or to attain certification in their fields; they also need to be able to find information to support their teaching of others, from health activity promotions to speaking engagements.

ANALYZING PATIENT OUTCOMES

Nurses may use evidence-based practices to support much of their work in clinical settings. When evaluating patient outcomes, research results of evidence-based practice can guide nurses toward determining what standards are working and what must be changed to develop the best outcomes for patients. Nurses may determine the need for change in practice as it affects patient outcomes. They may then **analyze evidence** targeted at the needed change to assess what can be applied to their current situation. If policies must be changed to implement the practice, a trial of practicing new methods may be necessary before actual policies are changed. If the practice benefits patient outcomes, it can then be implemented into regular standards of care. Finally, nurses must evaluate how well the evidence-based practice methods support patient outcomes after a period of time.

CLINICAL ARTICLES

There are several types of articles that nurses may publish as information for other nurses, including research outcomes, clinical articles, or articles related to evidence-based practice. **Clinical articles** are designed to disseminate information about clinical practice, in an attempt to improve care or promote debate about the topic. Clinical articles may give information about evidence-based practices that can be implemented; they may also cover topics, such as professional advancement, or they may be designed to discuss current concepts or controversies that are plaguing the nursing workforce. These articles are often published in nursing journals, as well as in online magazines, nursing newsletters, or books. Clinical articles are designed to be published, providing thoughts and ideas about how practices can be improved.

CHANGE CHAMPION

A **change champion** is a person who is familiar with evidence-based practice outcomes and works to communicate this information to involved staff. Often, change champions are individuals who work within the group, such as staff nurses or clinical nurse specialists. They review evidence about practices, including research results and expert opinions, and then develop educational settings where the information is given to staff to implement. Change champions use several different methods that may best facilitate change, depending on the situation and the receptivity of listeners. They are passionate about the topic and want others to know how it can benefit practice standards.

They are persistent and willing to communicate with others on many different levels to get their message across.

METHODS OF COMMUNICATING BEST PRACTICES

Communication is essential to educate others about the importance of evidence-based practices and their methods of use. Education may be provided through such measures as seminars for staff as part of learning; media coverage, including radio, television, or social networking; or small-group meetings to discuss the information. Small groups can allow discussion of the evidence and review possible practice changes. Small groups also give staff opportunities to voice their opinions about whether they want to implement changes or not. Communication methods that involve the exchange of ideas and interactive processing are often more effective at educating others about evidence-based practices than direct lectures or presentations.

IMPLEMENTING EVIDENCE-BASED INTERVENTIONS

Implementing evidence-based practices and changing methods of practice may not always be easy to do. In some cases, there can be more than one group promoting their evidence-based results, which may conflict. Some clinicians do not have time outside of patient care to perform literature reviews for evidence-based interventions and then apply them to patient care. Similarly, there may be nurses and practitioners who want to implement new changes, but do not understand how. Finally, some clinicians are slow to implement changes, even if the new methods are regarded as the new standard of care or best practice.

TRADITIONAL PRACTICES

Traditional nursing practices often follow standards that have been in place for generations, as older nurses impart the wisdom of certain techniques by saying simply "This is the way it is done." While these techniques and strategies may be historically the way things were done, they may not be based on sound clinical theory. When nurses follow traditional practices based on consensus from the unit, how they were taught in school, or how others always do it, they do not consider patients as individuals. Evidence-based practices provide updated and more concise information about certain practice standards that may replace many traditional practices; these evidence-based practices are designed to individualize patient care, provide nursing care that is focused on quality and problem-solving, and are effective in meeting patient outcomes.

TRIAL AND ERROR

In some situations where clear guidelines are not available, nurses may institute **trial and error** measures to devise effective methods of meeting patients' needs. For example, a clinical unit may have a patient with a unique condition that has little evidence in the literature for practice measures. Nurses may need to institute some trial and error measures, as long as they do not put the patient at risk to identify the best methods that meet the patient's needs. In most cases, however, trial and error measures provide more risk than they are worth as they are not based on sound evidence-based practices. They may waste valuable time and energy that could be used for other activities, and they may not be the best measures for the patient's condition. Additionally, when practices are not backed by research or policy, patients are put at risk of adverse outcomes.

BARRIERS TO EVIDENCE-BASED PRACTICE

When attempting to use evidence-based practices, nurses may encounter many **barriers** that prevent them from performing literature reviews, reading and discussing results, disseminating information, and adopting practices. Some barriers are time, lack of knowledge, or a lack of resources. There are several strategies nurses can adopt to counteract these barriers and make use of evidence-based practices a priority. Nurses can set aside a certain amount of time each month to

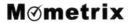

focus on reading research and performing literature reviews. If nurses do not know how to find literature, they can ask a librarian in a medical library for assistance. Nurses can take educational courses or seminars to learn more about the importance of evidence-based practices and performing literature searches. They may develop teams who work together to disseminate information gained through study. Finally, nurses may talk with others skilled in using evidence-based practices to learn more about the process.

Healthcare Finance and Economics

HEALTH CARE ECONOMIC CONCEPTS
RETURN ON INVESTMENT

Return on investment (ROI) is a method used to determine profitability, expressed as a percentage. The basic formula is:

- Net profit/total cost of investment X 100.

Thus, if an investment of $120,000 resulted in $200,000 in net profit:

- $200,000/$120,000 = 1.66 X 100 = 167% ROI.

Hospitals often run a narrow profit margin (2% average). Because of this, projected ROI is often calculated prior to investment. For example, if the hospital is considering investing in new equipment, profits would be projected over the expected life of the equipment, and costs for the equipment, maintenance, training, and upgrades would be estimated to determine if the ROI were favorable. The productivity advantage of equipment must also be calculated, based on yearly cost for employees utilizing the equipment, percentage of time they will use the equipment, percentage of estimated increased efficiency, and equipment training costs. Additionally, some types of programs, such as a community preventative program to identify and treat hypertension, may generate a negative ROI if complications and hospitalizations associated with hypertension reduce.

BUNDLED PAYMENTS

With **bundled payments** (AKA episode-of-care payments), payments are received by health care providers in a lump sum in advance of care for specific conditions or courses of treatment. This allows health care providers to focus on the patient's plan of care rather than reimbursement. The better the patient outcomes, the better the health care profit because every complication adds to cost of care. Bundled payments may cover multiple services and service providers.

VALUE-BASED PURCHASING

With **value-based purchasing**, a CMS program, the base MS-DRG payment is reduced by 2%, and acute hospitals receive incentive payments based on the quality of care in 4 domains: safety, clinical care, efficiency and cost reduction, and patient and caregiver-centered experience of care/care coordination. Hospitals are assigned improvement points depending on how far above or below they fall on the 50% benchmark established by the average scores of the top 10% of hospitals during the baseline period. Hospitals are also assigned consistency points by comparing hospital HCAHPS survey results to those of all hospitals surveyed. Based on these points, a total performance score is generated and VBP incentive payment determined.

BASIC MARKETING STRATEGIES

Basic marketing strategies employed in health care include:

- **Internal review:** Determining what unique characteristics the organization has that can provide an advantage over other organizations. This includes measurements across all aspects of the organization to determine current status in relation to other organizations.
- **External review/Market analysis:** Assessing community needs and determining where deficits occur to identify opportunities for provision of additional services. Determining the organization's market and resources as well as any obstacles the organization faces.
- **Growth initiatives:** Planning should look at opportunities for expansion, addition of staff, and addition of services.
- **Cost-benefit analysis:** Services, supplies, and equipment should be assessed in terms of return on investment, and cost-cutting measures taken where they do not impact the quality of service, such as buying in bulk and using different vendors.
- **Planning:** The organization should develop a comprehensive plan for the future and the direction the organization wants to take.

MARKET-BASED SYSTEM OF HEALTH CARE FINANCING

A **market-based system of health care financing** is that which is used in the United States for payment of health care services. In market-based financing, private industry pays for some of the costs of health care, such as through medical insurance companies. In other areas, the government also covers some costs for those who are classified as low-income, over a specific age, or disabled. This system of financing does provide medical coverage for those who can afford to pay premiums or those who receive government assistance. Those who do not meet the requirements for either private or government coverage, however, may go without benefits or the ability to pay for health care costs because they might have to pay out of pocket. Many people have jobs and low incomes, but their pay is not considered low enough to be considered for Medicaid. Additionally, because the government pays for some of the costs of care, Medicare and Medicaid programs can choose what costs they are willing to cover or deny.

COST ANALYSIS

Cost analysis refers to measuring the costs that are required to provide certain services. Within nursing, cost analysis considers each aspect of the health care environment to determine its costs and links it to the overall budget of running the environment. Costs in health care are broken down into different areas, depending on their purpose, function, and necessity. Some production costs that may be found within health care include cost of staffing, which involves paying salaries and benefits to nurses and other staff; the cost of materials used, such as medical instruments, health care technology, or nursing care supplies; the cost of facility expenses, such as utility bills, maintenance, cleaning, and use; and the cost of consumer satisfaction, by providing those aspects that will drive patients to return to the same health care institution, such as advertising, food, gifts, and educational campaigns.

CALCULATING COST-EFFECTIVENESS

Calculating costs of nursing interventions is important to determine if interventions are not only practical and helpful toward reaching patient outcomes but also **cost-effective**. Nursing interventions that are not cost-effective should be replaced by other interventions that are more cost-effective and still successful for patients. To determine the cost-effectiveness of a nursing intervention, nurses need to consider the cost of the intervention to begin with and divide it by the cost of the benefits for patients. This might not only be measured in numbers, but in other terms as well, such as how well patients respond to certain interventions as evidenced by reduction in disease symptoms, eradication of malignancy, or management of mental illness. Nurses, together with management, must assess whether the interventions they are providing are worth the time, money, and care to achieve positive patient outcomes.

RESOURCE UTILIZATION

Resource utilization involves considering what resources are available in the clinical setting, their cost-effectiveness, and how they affect nursing care and interventions. Nurses who consider the appropriate use of resources practice efficiently and economically, rather than wastefully. By practicing resource utilization, nurses consider what is available and use the systems that are most cost-effective while still providing adequate care. They also help patients and families to find resources that will meet their needs for care after discharge from the health organization. Nurses educate patients about cost-effectiveness of resources, how to learn more information about specific conditions and treatments, and how to determine the benefits and disadvantages of care. Finally, nurses who effectively practice resource utilization delegate responsibility, giving tasks only to those who are qualified to save time and resources for them to complete other tasks.

COST-EFFECTIVE CARE

Nurse-led initiatives provide quality care that is cost-effective for consumers who may often struggle with paying for health care services because of being uninsured or underinsured. Nurse-led initiatives also provide cost-effective care that serves the health care organization's budget as well. Clinics and health care units that employ nurse practitioners as part of their staff may save money because payment for these services is less than that for physicians. Nurse-managed clinics often provide preventive care services that may reduce the incidence of disease, thereby reducing overall health care costs for large populations. Other nurse-led programs, such as visiting nurses, educational programs, or research initiatives result in cost-savings through education of the community, greater adherence to treatment regimens, and more appropriate use of health care services.

PROMOTION OF NURSING EDUCATION

Recent **promotion of nursing education** to the baccalaureate level can help to improve the overall quality of nursing care practices and decrease associated risks, which may result in cost-effective care. When nurses receive advanced education, such as at the baccalaureate or master's levels, they learn more information beyond basic nursing care. Advanced nursing education focuses on leadership, research, finance, practice standards, and risk assessment, which are all subjects that nurses can consider while providing clinical care. When these subjects are taught, they may be more likely to be implemented into practice, thereby increasing quality of care in greater measures. These practices then may result in cost-effective measures, such as greater adherence to budget guidelines, more research that promotes cost-saving measures, introducing practice standards that reduce waste, and use of technology to make care more efficient, which also saves money for the organization.

EVALUATING COST-EFFECTIVENESS

Nursing services are essential components of health care, but managers and nurse leaders must often make decisions about how many nurses to employ. Adding nurses to a clinical unit is more costly than simply providing an annual salary. Many organizations are moving away from hiring more registered nurses and choosing to employ unlicensed assistive personnel as part of cost-saving measures. However, these personnel lack the education and expertise often needed in clinical situations for adequate patient care. Registered nurses provide a level of quality care that is unmatched by other positions requiring less education and training. Alternatively, health care payers may want to spend money on other programs, such as preventive services, wellness programs, and community education, instead of allocating their financial resources for paying nursing salaries. In each situation, the benefits of nursing care must outweigh the costs of its provision to keep registered nurses in the clinical care setting.

DISEASE PREVENTION ECONOMIC BENEFITS

Many health care organizations are focused on treatment of disease, and their money is spent accordingly; however, **prevention of disease** can provide many economic benefits for society and is becoming a greater focus among providers seeking to reduce costs. Disease prevention benefits society through lowering overall health care costs, such as by controlling diseases so that fewer treatments are needed; reducing obesity, stress, or smoking, that contribute to multiple high-cost complications; and decreasing the inappropriate use of facilities for health care, such as use of emergency rooms for minor illness outbreaks. Prevention also provides benefits because it increases the productivity of workers by reducing injuries, promoting healthy lifestyles, and reducing absenteeism.

HEALTH INFORMATION TECHNOLOGY

Health information technology (IT) is designed to improve overall functioning within the health care system by implementing and managing technology within the health care environment. This technology improves the safety of patients, streamlines many nursing responsibilities, and increases quality measures of nursing care. Health care IT may reduce health care costs through these measures. When the safety of patients is guarded through IT, such as through tracking systems for sentinel events or monitoring of risk factors, overall costs may be reduced with the reduction in costly errors. By streamlining nursing care, such as through electronic health records, IT helps to make nursing care more efficient, which reduces costs in labor. Health care IT also improves costs by recognizing and tracking quality measures. When health care units embrace quality, the organization runs more efficiently and remains up to standards set by such organizations as the Joint Commission. Costs that might have been incurred to pay fines for not keeping quality measures in place are also reduced.

PRODUCT SELECTION PROCESS

Nurses who are part of **product selection** may participate in many decisions about what products to buy for the organization, which may then be used in clinical practice. Before making a decision based only on item cost and quality of use, nurses must evaluate the company providing the product to determine the expected level of support for using the product. Nurses may check with clinicians at other organizations to determine their level of success with using the product or any negative opinions about it. If the product is new, nurses might need to find out if the company providing the product offers education for staff about how to use it. They should know if the product has a warranty, who to contact if there are further questions, or if installation of the product is necessary.

HOSPITAL PRODUCT-EVALUATION COMMITTEE

A **product-evaluation committee** is comprised of members of an organization who review and evaluate products used in the organization to determine how cost-effective they are. The work of the product-evaluation committee has an effect on the financial aspects of using certain products by determining their associated expenses; identifying other products that are less expensive, which can be substituted; determining whether some products can be reused or recycled; changing practices that are costly; determining where practices can be changed or eliminated to reduce costs; determining whether the organization could order less to save money; or performing a budget analysis to determine if new products can be implemented.

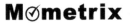

NURSES AND ECONOMISTS

Nurses and **economists** have many overlapping goals when the topic is best practices for patient outcomes. By working together on an interdisciplinary team, nurses and economists can facilitate appropriate care that is cost-effective and promotes positive outcomes for patients. Nurses have insight into what patients need through interventions, and economists can take examples of these interventions to determine their cost-effectiveness. Additionally, nurses and economists may work together to determine how the working environment may be more efficient and cost-effective without sacrificing quality for patient outcomes. Working together, nurses and economists may be able to strategize ideas for managing nursing shortages in some locations as well as develop cost-effective measures for retaining the nursing staff that is available.

INTANGIBLE ASSETS

When determining the **financial value of assets** within a health care organization, there may be tangible or intangible assets to consider.

- **Tangible assets** comprise the physical items used for health care as well as the building where the organization is housed.
- **Intangible assets** may be harder to recognize, but still must be considered when determining the financial value of an organization and implementation into the budget. Examples of intangible assets include the skills of nursing staff, relationships between the organization and consumers, health care agreements, medical records, regulatory approvals, franchise rights, computer software and information technology, or historical documents related to the organization.

BENCHMARKING COSTS

Benchmarking is an ongoing process of measuring practice, outcomes, and services against a standard. External benchmarking involves analyzing data from outside an organization. In order for this data to be meaningful, the same definitions must be used in comparison as well as the same populations or effective risk stratification. Using national data can be informative, but each institution is different, and relying on only external benchmarking to select indicators for processes can be misleading. Widespread research and careful data analysis are necessary to identify high cost/high volume activities when establishing benchmarks nationally and across care settings. These data can help provide guidance for making health care policy and can provide information about the quality and costs of health care to help consumers make informed decisions. Benchmarking can help organizations to manage costs, as one budget goal should be to match benchmarks and to reward doing so.

VALUATION

Valuation describes the process of identifying the worth of certain resources within a company. Within health care, valuation of nursing requires that organizations define the worth of nursing staff as resources compared with the costs of maintaining these services with other personnel. When a valuation study is performed to determine the value of nursing care, organizations are better able to determine what assets they have available in both nursing care and tangible resources. Additionally, a valuation study justifies the nurses employed and payment for their services, as well as the need to employ more nurses to maintain standards and levels of quality. A valuation study also helps health care organizations to prove to shareholders and third-party payers the worth of staff employed as well as the worth of the organization.

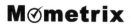

SEPARATING NURSING COSTS FROM STANDARD HOSPITAL CHARGES

In most billing systems of health care organizations, nursing care costs are combined as part of the charges for hospital use and room charges. Hospitals are paid based on a set fee for charges accrued while staying in a hospital bed within a certain unit. This does not account for the acuity of nursing care provided. **Separating nursing care costs** from room charges in hospitals may help nurse–patient ratios if nurses are paid according to the care provided. It may decrease the workload that nurses carry because of downsizing in other areas designed to cut costs. Nurses would also have a greater understanding of the economic impact of their roles, in terms of time, materials, and hospital assets.

STEWARDSHIP

Stewardship involves using available resources, making the best of them, and planning for the future to continue to improve standards. Nurses can be good stewards of their financial resources by minimizing waste by using supplies accordingly. They are obligated to consider the budget for the nursing unit to determine where reductions can be made in supply costs. They should consider the cost-effectiveness of nursing interventions as related to patient outcomes. They can take care of the technology, supplies, and materials with which they currently work to prevent further costs in repairs. Nurses should also consider the financial department of the organization where they work to learn more about fiscal management, as this department can provide great insight about overall costs of running a health care business.

PURCHASING COMMITTEE

Some organizations have a purchasing department in which a few select people decide what items and products are used as part of patient care. There are other organizations, though, where a **purchasing committee** works together as a multidisciplinary team to evaluate products and decide which ones are the best fit for patient care. Nurses are important members of these purchasing committees because they have a first-hand understanding of the value and feasibility of some products, but they can also relay information about items that do not work as well. Nurses who want to become involved in purchasing may volunteer to serve on the purchasing committee to evaluate products and become involved in their purchase and implementation. The purchasing committee may also consist of other workers in the organization, such as maintenance, bioengineering, fiscal employees, or physicians, who all have a stake in what items are purchased.

FISCAL RESPONSIBILITIES

Fiscal responsibility is part of the role of nurses as leaders, and yet many nurse leaders are uneducated and unprepared to handle fiscal responsibilities. Most nurses have received training in patient care and even management, but they often have received little educational preparation in finance; thus, some nurses are unaware of the financial impact of their jobs and do not focus on fiscal responsibility. There are also some nurses who do not believe that economics is a part of nursing responsibilities and would rather focus on direct patient care. Nurses who are promoted into leadership or management positions may be responsible for some fiscal directives but have never actually been trained in these matters. Finally, there are some nurses who are unfamiliar with the language of fiscal terms and do not understand financial matters at all; these nurses may have an extremely difficult time trying to incorporate fiscal responsibility into their jobs.

MEDICARE REIMBURSEMENT

When patients receive **Medicare** services and must have hospital care, Medicare typically pays a set amount of money for certain services to the health care facility. This amount has been predetermined and may or may not cover the actual cost of services for the patient. The set amount also does not consider where the patient lives in the United States and if health care costs for certain procedures are higher in some areas than in others. Medicare develops the payment amount based on what it considers to be a reasonable rate for procedures and treatments and then pays accordingly. If a condition develops during hospitalization and increases a patient's length of stay, such as ventilator-associated pneumonia, Medicare often will not pay for the additional care that is necessary.

HEALTH INSURANCE COVERAGE

Health insurance coverage is often confusing for patients who must sort through the information provided to determine what is covered and for what they must pay. Nurses may be able to assist patients with determining what services are covered under their health care policies based on information provided. Many insurance documents provide information about covered services as compared to those that are denied. Some services must have proven benefits, in that they are medically sound and not investigational in order to be covered. Other procedures must be deemed medically necessary according to policy. There are also some situations in which exclusions apply, and the patient should understand what these might be. For instance, some health insurance companies do not pay for cosmetic surgeries or those that are not deemed essential to maintain health and prevent disease.

LACK OF HEALTH INSURANCE

There are millions of people in the United States who do not have **access** to adequate health insurance. In many cases, people are underinsured, while millions more have no insurance at all. State health insurance programs cover some care for children, and Medicaid is an option for some, but many providers refuse to take some patients because of low reimbursement amounts. Lack of health insurance results in poor care management on the part of patients, who either do not know where to go for care or cannot afford care when they need it. This may increase the spread of disease, the complications of chronic diseases, and mortality. It also results in inappropriate use of facilities when uninsured patients seek non-emergent care in hospital emergency departments.

HEALTH CARE FINANCING

Health care financing refers to the systems by which health care is funded, and the type of health care financing available to people has a profound impact on access to care because of prohibitive health care costs. In the United States, systems include: government funded (Medicare, Medicaid, Children's Health Insurance Plan, VA), private insurance (Blue Cross®, Blue Shield®), self-payment, and volunteer/donated aid (Shriner's Hospitals). Patients on Medicare (which pays 80% of costs) but without supplemental insurance may still face huge bills. Additionally, many physicians no longer accept Medicare/Medicaid patients, limiting access. Patients with no medical coverage, such as those who are ineligible for Medicare/Medicaid but can't afford private insurance, often have very limited access to physicians and may be unable to afford treatment or medications. Health care is often neglected, resulting in chronic illness, pain, disability, and complications that might have been avoided with adequate care.

FINANCIALLY RELATED ETHICAL ISSUES

Nurses are required to follow a code of conduct in practice, although there may be some situations in which guidelines are not clearly defined. **Ethical issues** may occur when nurses are in situations in which they must make a choice between what they feel is right or wrong. Nurses may encounter financial issues within their practices that require ethical decision-making as well. There are multiple examples available that might describe this phenomenon, including managed care, which might be focused on increasing quality of patient care, but there might also be cost-cutting measures and decreased revenue. Some health care organizations are making cuts in the workforce of registered nurses to employ unlicensed assistive personnel to save money. Health care providers may limit diagnostic testing or treatments because of decreased payments from health maintenance organizations or preferred provider organizations.

FEDERAL ANTI-KICKBACK STATUTE

The **federal Anti-Kickback Statute** makes it illegal for health care organizations to accept money or rewards from sources as a method of getting them to use certain services. For example, a hospital unit cannot accept gifts or money from a certain health care provider in the community if it makes more referrals to the specific provider. There are some situations, called "Safe Harbors," which may appear to violate the Anti-Kickback Statute but are still allowable under law. For example, some companies can provide discounted services for certain providers or medications, as long as the patients involved are informed of the situation and the information is fully documented.

Healthcare Informatics

HEALTH INFORMATICS AND HEALTH INFORMATION MANAGEMENT

Both health informatics and health information management are systems that seek to manage health information.

- **Health informatics** involves the use of computer technology to design, organize, and implement patient care; collect and store data; track and analyze trends; and create reports that lead to change in health practices. Health informatics allows for communication among providers, using a streamlined process of patient care to provide efficiency and quality.
- **Health information management** also involves the organization of data and communication among providers, but this field is centered on individual information, such as medical records of patients, diagnostic groups, or billing codes.

HEALTH AND WELLNESS TOPICS INTERNET RESEARCH

The **internet** provdes access to a wealth of information for patients and families who are seeking advice or data about their health or diseases. Patients are able to search easily and find information on a variety of health topics, which may then give further direction as to how to manage care, find treatments, or make other decisions. For people who have internet access, they can stay up-to-date on current treatments, join forums to share with people who have similar conditions, or read data about their medications. Alternatively, there may be incorrect information at certain internet sites. Patients may believe that they are finding valuable information when in fact they may be reading material that has been written by individuals without the appropriate background in the field.

DETERMINING CREDIBILITY OF A HEALTH WEBSITE

There are websites that help nurses to find important information about health and wellness; however, many websites contain inaccurate information, personal opinions, or targeted agendas. Nurses must learn to distinguish whether or not a health-information website is credible. One simple way to do so is to consider the domain that is hosting the information. For example, a url that ends with .gov is a government website and one that ends with .edu is an educational institution, both of which are typically credible. Nurses should also look for an author's name and credentials associated with the site or information. Nurses should look at advertising on the website and its topics to see if it is associated with the focus of the webpage or something else. Finally, nurses should determine when the information on the website was written by searching for a date of publication. Old material may continue to be available long after it has become inaccurate if the webpage is not updated regularly.

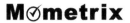

EDUCATING PATIENTS ABOUT INTERNET USE

Many patients are more informed about their health after accessing websites for information. They may already know a lot of information before stepping into a health care organization. Unfortunately, many websites are not credible, and some patients may find misleading information. Nurses can educate patients about using the internet by teaching them that they should be careful where they look. Nurses can tell patients about the type of sites for which to look by considering domain names, the name and title of the author, and advertising on the site. Nurses can advise patients to avoid blogs or articles of personal opinion that might have little basis in fact. Nurses might provide patients with links to sites with valuable health information; they can also direct patients to use a public or medical library, which may reduce the number of sites to credible and verified sources.

TECHNOLOGY

Technology is designed to streamline many processes in nursing care and to minimize those extra steps that may otherwise be necessary. **Incorporating technology** improves the clinical care delivery process by making certain processes more efficient, such as documentation, transferring of documents, or recording important data. Nurses may be able to communicate more efficiently with providers and other caregivers with technology. The clinical environment may be safer and give patients more quality care because data are organized and then added to existing knowledge bases to improve practice. Nurses may use technology to educate their patients through certain delivery systems or for access to information that they can be easily forwarded. Finally, technology allows nurses to monitor patients' vital signs and other important health data to be analyzed over a period of time.

NURSING INFORMATICS

Nursing informatics is a comprehensive system that combines nursing, computer science, and health information management into a method of monitoring patient care outcomes, communicating among providers, and evaluating the effectiveness of interventions. Informatics uses electronic medical records (EHRs), computerized charting systems, and patient monitoring systems to keep track of patients' needs while they are receiving care. These systems allow nurses to design patient outcomes through such measures as providing health information at a glance or offering templates to organize patient outcomes for certain situations. Nurses also use informatics to evaluate the effectiveness of health outcomes through monitoring systems that tell nurses the health status of patients; electronic documentation, which allows nurses to chart and track patient trends as they move toward stated goals; and EHRs, which allow comparisons between patients' current conditions and past records of health outcomes.

ELECTRONIC HEALTH RECORDS

Electronic health records (EHRs) are being implemented into more facilities, and many clinicians are aware of the benefits of using this type of documentation. The EHRs not only improve the speed and effectiveness of documentation, but providers can use EHRs to communicate with each other regarding certain patients in a way that can save much time. The EHRs also contribute to quality patient outcomes by their capabilities for maintaining and analyzing information. For example, if a patient takes a specific medication, the EHR may flag the account if information is entered regarding a new prescription for the patient who will react negatively to the current medication. The EHRs maintained in certain locations allow providers to access patient information quickly upon return to their offices. Finally, EHRs can track errors that would normally be too difficult to identify or trail through a paper-based system.

POINT OF CARE

Nurses have increased access to technologies that may be used at the **point of care** to guide them in their work, to communicate with physicians, and to increase the speed of documentation. Point-of-care technologies may range from personal digital assistants that nurses can keep at the bedside to notebook computers that allow nurses to identify and document information without leaving the patient's side. Point-of-care technology often frees nurses to focus on patients, their needs, and their current health status to monitor for changes or to provide education. It provides nurses with quick access to patient statistics, such as health history, medications, or allergies. It allows nurses to communicate with physicians, often with the patient right next to them, to ensure that they communicate accurate and timely data that will help patients. Finally, nursing point-of-care technology may perform various tasks that analyze or explain data about patients, such as disease processes, responses to certain medications, or even financial figures.

Patient Care Technology

CLINICAL INFORMATION SYSTEMS
SELECTING OF A CLINICAL INFORMATION SYSTEM

When a health care organization decides to integrate a new clinical information system into its processes or upgrade its current system, at least one member of the nursing staff should be involved in the decision-making process. Because nurses are at the frontline of patient care, their input and expertise are invaluable in the selection of a new system. They can provide perspectives about important issues, concerns, and daily management of systems because they are typically the most common users of the systems. Their use of the systems directly affects patient care, which they are responsible for delivering. Nurses are in a position to provide input about the safety, ease of use, quality, and feasibility of electronic health systems.

CONSIDERATIONS WHEN EVALUATING EFFECTIVENESS

Because nurses often use **electronic information systems** as part of patient care and dissemination of information, it is important that they understand the essential components of these systems, not only to use them accurately but also to offer insight if changes are made. Evaluation of systems involves considering the documentation process and how efficient it is for nurses to record patient information; for instance, some documentation may be recorded in real time, while other systems may allow nurses to return later to add important information. Ease of use is another critical component, as most nurses do not have time to maneuver through multiple screens to search for place at which to record important information. Systems should be easily accessible and usable to provide more time for patient care. The system's ability to transmit information should be considered, not only for its capabilities but also for the protection of confidential patient information. Finally, the system should be reliable, in that it works consistently and has technical support available should problems arise.

WIRELESS PATIENT-MONITORING SYSTEM

Wireless monitoring systems are designed to record patient data, such as vital signs or oxygen levels in a continuous manner, while allowing nurses to leave the patient's bedside. The systems are used so that nurses can move between patients while still monitoring their vital information. If a patient's condition changes, the nurse is notified through a wireless system, such as a pager. Wireless systems offer convenience for nurses who are caring for several patients at once, some of whom may be very ill, and need to leave the bedside. Wireless monitoring systems are also designed to save time for nurses who spend their time looking for equipment, monitoring patients, and seeking out other nurses, Alternatively, without the nurse at the bedside, patients may be at

116

high risk of falling if they try to get up without assistance. There may also be a greater length of time between adverse events and providing rescue than if nurses were nearby and not dependent on a wireless system.

COMPUTERIZED PROVIDER ORDER ENTRY

A **computerized provider order entry (CPOE)** is the process of ordering medications for patients through a computer system that automatically transmits the information to the pharmacy that dispenses the medication. A CPOE streamlines the process whereby physicians write out orders, the order is transcribed, the pharmacy fills the order, and the nurse dispenses the medication. The benefits of a CPOE are that pharmacists and nurses do not have to decipher illegible writing that often accompanies certain prescriptions. Physicians may choose a set dosage or type of medication, which makes the ordering process more efficient. The CPOE almost eliminates the need for transcribing the order, which saves time and reduces mistakes. Nurses are much less likely to make errors when administering medication when the prescription is computerized.

NURSING INFORMATION SYSTEM

A **nursing information system** is a special component of health care that combines information technology with nursing care. Nursing information systems are programs that manage patient data and communicate important information to nurses caring for patients. The data may come from several areas within the organization and may then be organized into a useful framework that can be implemented by nurses. Some ways in which nursing information systems may be used include electronic health record documentation, scheduling of nursing shifts, tracking of disease progression to assist clinicians with making health care decisions, or combining information from several disciplines to individualize patient-care standards.

FORMULATING DIAGNOSES

Nurses may use health care technologies to help them with performing the nursing process, including formulating **nursing diagnoses**. Health care technology may assist nurses with the assessment phase of the nursing process; nurses use technology to perform such assessments as vital signs, evaluating symptoms, or taking patients' histories. This information may be stored in an electronic health record to provide a complete picture of the patients' health. Nurses can use this information to determine applicable nursing diagnoses for patients' conditions, which will help guide interventions and formulate outcomes. Some software programs track information input and formulate nursing diagnoses for nurses. Through technology, nurses can also track their interventions aimed at supporting nursing diagnoses.

TELEMEDICINE

At one time, **telemedicine** involved the use of a landline telephone between a patient and a nurse to assess the patient's condition. While this method is still in use today, there are also many new technologies that nurses employ to assess patients through telemedicine. Patients can access nursing care through online services on their computers or through Smart televisions to have face-to-face interactions. Other sources, such as remote monitoring devices, track patient information and allow nurses to monitor patients from a distance. These devices allow nurses to see patients' vital signs and oxygenation levels even when they are not physically next to them. Technology called store and forward techniques take in patient information where it is stored for nurses to access later. This technology allows nurses in telemedicine to look back over past information of their patients to analyze trends and to make decisions for the next step in their patients' plan of care.

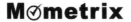

WORK-FLOW TECHNOLOGY

A work-flow system streamlines the process of getting patients from one point of care to the next. **Work-flow technology** may be used to make the process of discharging patients from the health care environment more efficient. By using a work-flow system, nurses can alert those needed to take the next step of getting patients home. Nurses may use the system to notify transport to pick up patients and take them to their car, for example; environmental services may be notified to come and clean the room, and the nursing supervisor can be notified that the bed is ready and available for the next patient. This system reduces the amount of time nurses have to spend making phone calls and communicating with departments to determine if they are doing their jobs and if patients are safely discharged home.

TECHNOLOGY TO MANAGE WOUND CARE

Wound care management is required in many health care settings, from long-term care facilities to acute health care settings. Nurses must not only understand how to manage wounds when they develop, but they must know the potential causes of wound development to facilitate better prevention. Nursing technology can manage wound care by tracking those patients who may be more likely to develop wounds, such as bedridden patients or those with diabetes. Technology involves the use of certain types of beds or measures to reduce pressure on the skin. Wound-management technology may also consist of monitoring systems that can check patients' circulation, as well as follow the progress of their wounds to determine whether they are worsening. Finally, technological innovations also allow for tracking and documenting consults, medications, and treatments that are all needed for managing patients' wounds.

TECHNOLOGY FOR PAIN MANAGEMENT

Physicians and nurses are able to incorporate technology into assessing, managing, and treating **pain** in their patients in remarkable ways. Providers who use mobile devices have specific apps available that help to calculate medication dosages, flag side effects and interactions, and have quick access to medication references. Physicians also have access to many technological devices that are designed specifically for treatment or control of pain, such as electrotherapy, use of infrared heat, joint stimulators, and radiofrequency equipment, in addition to prescribing pain medications. Additionally, the electronic medical record can record, track, and analyze pain management interventions to assess what is successful and what must be changed.

COMBATING INFECTION

Besides hand washing, disinfecting, and following manual infection control procedures, there are some **technologies that can combat infections** in some health care organizations. Some technologies use high-intensity ultraviolet light to kill pathogens and microorganisms in the air and on surfaces in rooms. Some programs are using new equipment in patients' rooms that are resistant to bacteria that can contribute to infections. Computerized educational programs provide simulation experiences so that nurses can identify situations that may cause infections with no risk to patients, but practitioners still introduce measures as to how to respond. Finally, many software systems are used in health care organizations that review documentation of patient care and can direct providers about interventions that will prevent infection, even going so far as to send alerts about certain interventions.

MEDICAL INFORMATION SOFTWARE

Medical information software is important for the **billing process** for patients to pay for their health care services. If patients have medical coverage through health insurance, nurses or billing specialists must determine this at the beginning of the visit. When patients receive services, the

118

diagnosis and the treatment measures are coded to determine how much will be covered. Codes are assigned for treatments, procedures, tests, or surgery. Certain charges are associated with each code. In many ways, the software used for billing is an accounting method that measures the charges coded for each procedure to determine how much to bill the insurance company or to charge the patient.

GROUPWARE

Groupware is a type of computer technology that uses computer network systems for collaborating between members of teams or groups that are working on similar strategies. Because groups must work together to achieve their goals, groupware facilitates communication to work toward these goals and to promote progress. It is often used through the internet. Groupware is successful because it coordinates communication between team members, even when they are not directly present for the meeting. It can save money for those who have to travel to meet with the group by allowing them to meet via distance technology, and it allows team members to exchange ideas, thereby facilitating increased exchange of perspectives for critical situations.

COMPUTER-MEDIATED COMMUNICATION

Within nursing, **computer-mediated communication (CMC)** provides communication among nurses, among nurses and providers, or other members of the interdisciplinary team. Use of CMC may be through video messaging or instant messaging, which allows users to work on teams across distances. Text messaging is another form of CMC, which provides fast results or orders for interventions. Other methods of CMC may help nurses to communicate about treatment plans, specific disease symptoms and management, cultural variables, quality measures, or staffing issues. The use of CMC not only provides knowledge and communication about essential nursing duties but also support and cooperation at times when they may be needed most.

COMMUNICATION TECHNOLOGIES

Nurses are required to perform a multitude of duties every day, and much of it is not direct patient care. Beyond bedside care, nurses must perform quality-improvement measures, organize plans of care, meet on interdisciplinary teams, and spend time documenting their work. New communication technology implemented into nursing practice can help **save time** that nurses spend being fixed at a desk or walking back and forth to answer pages. Wireless headsets allow nurses to answer calls while they are still in patients' rooms, if they need to be. Badges are available that can be clipped to nursing uniforms that allow others to quickly locate where nurses are at the moment, which reduces time that others must spend looking for them. Bedside computers allow nurses to search patients' results or document medications while still in the room. New communication technologies that save time in mundane tasks help to increase nurses' efficiency and allow them to spend more time with their patients

MEETING THE NEEDS OF CERTAIN COMMUNITIES

Technological advances have increased greatly in recent decades, providing accurate data, availability of tracking information, and rapid communication between providers. The electronic health record is one system that enables health care providers to document patient care as well as transmit this information between providers if necessary, to promote interdisciplinary care. Prescriptions and health forms can be electronically transmitted to provide quick answers about patients' conditions, thus potentially slowing lengths of stay. Health care providers also have greater access to electronic resources, such as the internet or information-storage sites, which allow them to look up pertinent information or communicate with other providers who are in similar situations. Finally, nurses may communicate on social networking sites if they work in

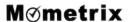

similar care situations. This may provide a level of camaraderie between professionals who share the joys and drawbacks of working in specific settings.

INSTRUCTIONAL TECHNOLOGY

Instructional technology is a process used to deliver educational information that is developed through planning, organizing, managing, using, and evaluating the resources available. Instructional technology develops instructional methods that are appropriate for the learners involved and uses these methods to deliver educational information in methods that are effective. In health care, instructional technology considers not only the educational needs of patients, but also their abilities to access the information and grasp the concepts. By recognizing these situations, instructional technology provides educational information through various means that will reach patients for their educational needs. For example, some patients are better visual learners and can grasp more health care information when it is presented as a video or demonstration. There are some patients who also benefit from reading materials that address information and need to be taught in this manner. Instructional technology provides opportunities for the presentation of information that will best meet the learning needs of patients.

INFORMATION ABOUT MEDICAL TECHNOLOGY

With the many advances in medical technology in the health care environment, patients may feel overwhelmed by the different technological measures available for their care. Nurses may need to **explain the purpose of this technology** so that patients understand what types of machines are being used in their care. Nurses can explain by using clear and simple language and avoiding complicated technical or medical jargon. Nurses should also talk about the benefits of using such technology and how it helps the patient, which instills greater faith in the measures and the organization.

TECHNOLOGY TO MINIMIZE ERRORS

Technology is designed to help nurses in their work by **reducing errors** and making the care environment a safer place for patients. There are several types of technology available that have been created to warn nurses of potentially hazardous situations, such as changes in patients' conditions or the potential for accidents. Some examples include alarms on intravenous (IV) pumps that warn of IV occlusions, wireless systems that notify nurses of patients' decreased oxygen levels, bed alarms that warn nurses if patients try to get out of bed without help, alarms on ventilators that signify decreased pressure, nurse-call systems that allow patients to call nurses for help, and bedside code buttons that allow nurses to press a button quickly for help if patients are deteriorating.

PERSONAL HEALTH RECORDS

Personal health records are electronic records where patients can keep track of their private health information to use when needed. Personal health records can be filled out and kept online, which can be accessed only by authorized users. Patients may keep a secured account and access the information on their own time to update it and make changes when necessary. If patients are admitted to the hospital or seek emergency care, physicians may access the personal health record with the patients' permission. This allows physicians to have quick access to the patients' health background and current medications. There are some software programs that provide personal health records, which allow patients to make appointments with providers, fill prescriptions, or send emails to providers about their conditions.

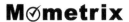

ELECTRONIC HEALTH RECORDS

Electronic documentation is slowly replacing paper-based files in health care organizations. There are several reasons why electronic health records (EHRs) are more efficient than paper-based systems. Files with papers may be difficult to decipher, particularly because charting is handwritten and may be illegible. Paper-based files are cumbersome and require much more room for storage than digital files. An EHR allows patient information to be easily disseminated among providers; alternatively, when patients have a paper-based file at one location, their records tend to stay there except through faxing, mailing, or other methods of sharing documents. EHRs can hold more information that can be accessed at a glance, rather than sifting through hundreds of documents that may be in various locations. Finally, EHRs allow providers to communicate with access to health histories that are comprehensive and complete, which may reduce the number of mistakes associated with incorrect information.

USE OF ELECTRONIC HEALTH RECORDS ON PATIENTS' PRIVACY

Upholding patients' **privacy** is an essential component of health care, as organizations must comply with the Health Information Portability and Accountability Act. This act requires health care organizations to follow the law related to protecting patient privacy by not sharing private health information about patients except with health care providers who are directly related to their care. The use of the electronic health records (EHRs) may blend some of these lines, as it may be difficult to control who accesses patients' records and for what purposes. The EHRs are valuable tools to not only electronically record information about patients but also to collaborate with other providers about patient care. When providers share information or when multiple sources have access to personal information for patients through the EHR, patients' privacy may be breached. Because of the electronic dissemination of information, it may be difficult to control who has access to records and who protects patients' privacy.

MEDICAL IDENTITY THEFT

Identity theft, in which a person's financial and other private information is breached, is very similar to medical identity theft, which involves a breach of private health information. Medical identity theft occurs when patients' health information is accessed, which often occurs through electronic health records (EHRs). Information about patients may be altered, so that the altered record affects treatment, prescriptions, or billing. Changed medical information may also result in fraudulent billing to insurance companies or Medicare for services not completed. Additionally, patients may have medical records that are inaccurate for their health care needs. For example, patients whose records have been changed due to medical identity theft may have several treatments recorded that never happened. When patients present for care, physicians could potentially order treatments based on inaccurate information.

TECHNOLOGY SECURITY TOOLS

Because electronic health records may be accessed inappropriately, technology security tools are put in place to protect private health information. **Security tools** are designed to ensure that only appropriate users gain access to private information through login requirements and encryption. They limit how much information even authorized users are allowed to access so that only pertinent information to the current situation is available. Security tools maintain updated information and send alerts or reminders about when security should be updated. They may also remind users to log off computers or may require users to provide authentication again after a certain period of use to determine that the appropriate person is using the information. They provide firewalls and other management services to prevent outside users from illegally accessing

121

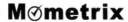

information. Finally, security tools can track or audit individuals who have accessed information about certain patients to determine whether the situation was appropriate.

ACCIDENTAL DISCLOSURES

Accidental disclosures are situations in which patients' privacy is breached unintentionally. This may occur in such situations as someone overhearing part of a conversation that was taking place in private or a health care worker stumbling upon private information about someone known personally. Accidental disclosures are typically innocent in nature but can still be prevented with appropriate security while using health technology. Nurses who access electronic medical records should only access records of their assigned patients and sign off their computers when finished. If nurses must walk away from a computer terminal, even for a minute or two, they should log off or minimize information on the screen so that it is not left in the open for anyone to see. Nurses should consider private information when leaving phone messages, sending faxes, or sending e-mails to ensure that unintended recipients do not accidentally get the information.

SOCIAL MEDIA

Social media are valuable tools for accessing information about health from credible sources as well as disseminating information. Nurses also use social networking to gather with others through forums or online groups to provide support. Social networking must be used carefully, as it may also invade the privacy of patients. Nurses should never provide information about patients through social networking sites. Additionally, nurses should be careful about what information they provide about themselves, as others can easily access this information to find pictures and personal information. Nurses should remember that they are professional employees of an organization and should not post information that would reflect negatively on the organization where they work.

CNL Practice Test

1. The hospital is shifting from paper records to electronic medical records (EMR), and the CNL is a member of the committee that has selected a vendor. Which of the following must be completed before a final selection can be made?

    a. Needs assessment.
    b. Financial plan.
    c. Staff training.
    d. Computer purchases.

2. Which of the following is the first step in ethical decision-making?

    a. Identify important/key participants.
    b. Identify options.
    c. Determine moral perspectives.
    d. Gather data.

3. The CNL notes an increased incidence of client injuries in a unit with Alzheimer patients. Which of the following BEST demonstrates that the CNL is competent at researching best practices for prevention of patient injuries?

    a. The CNL conducts a survey of staff opinions about prevention.
    b. The CNL makes observations in a facility with a low incidence of patient injuries.
    c. The CNL conducts systematic research utilizing online medical databases.
    d. The CNL utilizes clinical judgment to develop prevention measures.

4. A hospice client with metastatic pancreatic cancer has lost 50 pounds and now weighs only 102 pounds and is very cachectic with loss of adipose tissue and muscle wasting. The client's pain has been treated with fentanyl patches (50 mg), which are changed every 3 days, but the client's pain control is very poor, and she is taking one to two OxyContin (oxycodone) 5 mg tablets every 4 to 6 hours for breakthrough pain. A novice hospice nurse asks the CNL for advice about pain control. Which of the following is the BEST first action?

    a. Increase dosage of fentanyl patches.
    b. Increase dosage of OxyContin for breakthrough pain.
    c. Add an adjuvant medication, such as an NSAID.
    d. Switch from fentanyl patches to long-acting oral narcotic.

5. The CNL's primary responsibility is to provide leadership at

    a. Team conferences.
    b. Administrative meetings.
    c. Point of care.
    d. Discharge planning.

6. Which of the following actions by the CNL is part of the core CNL role of leadership?

    a. The CNL takes a course in oncologic pharmacology when assigned to an oncology unit.
    b. The CNL delegates client care to team members.
    c. The CNL calculates the cost-effectiveness of new procedures.
    d. The CNL uses evidence-based research to develop care plans.

7. The CNL must evaluate patient safety on a medical-surgical unit. The most effective initial method is to

    a. Interview staff individually.
    b. Conduct a staff survey with the AHRQ Hospital Survey on Patient Safety Culture.
    c. Conduct a patient survey regarding satisfaction with care.
    d. Establish a focus group.

8. The CNL is utilizing the PFA (purpose-focus-approach) method to develop an Internet search for materials for colleagues regarding best practices. Which type of search is most indicated?

    a. Broad, general search using key words.
    b. Lay-oriented search of non-technical sites, such as WebMD.
    c. Professionally oriented search of medical databases and professional organizations.
    d. Narrow technically oriented search with very specific parameters.

The following scenario applies to questions 9 and 10

As part of the promotion of a culture of safety, the organization has introduced a Just Culture approach. One of the nurses on the CNL's team needs to transfer an obese client from the bed to a wheelchair, and protocol calls for a two-person transfer. However, the nurse believes he can safely transfer the client alone since other staff members are occupied. The nurse begins the transfer, but the client panics and begins resisting, resulting in a fall to the floor. While x-rays show no fractures, the client is bruised and in pain.

9. How would this type of safety event be classified under the Just Culture model?

    a. Human error.
    b. At-risk behavior.
    c. Reckless behavior.
    d. Insubordinate behavior.

10. What type of response by the CNL is most appropriate under the Just Culture model?

    a. Consolation.
    b. Punitive action.
    c. Self-evaluation.
    d. Coaching.

11. The CNL has been chosen to represent nurses in collective bargaining. The management wants to maintain the status quo and give as little as possible while the union wants to maximize salary and benefit gains. If one side wins, the other side loses. This type of collective bargaining is

    a. Distributive.
    b. Integrative.
    c. Productivity.
    d. Composite.

12. During lunch with a team member, the team member tells the CNL she overheard a conversation between a client and his visitor and begins to share salacious gossip about the client's personal life. Which is the BEST response?

    a. Listen without responding.
    b. Change the subject.
    c. Confront the team member about violating professional ethics.
    d. Tell the team member he/she shouldn't tell anyone else.

13. A client with osteomyelitis had a PICC line inserted for long-term antibiotic therapy but developed sensitivity to the transparent dressing. Because the insertion site is now covered with a gauze dressing, the staff is unable to monitor the insertion site visually for signs of infection. Which of the following should the CNL recommend as the BEST safety measure to prevent infection?

    a. Change the gauze dressing every 24 hours to inspect the insertion site.
    b. Palpate the insertion site for tenderness daily. If no signs of infection, leave the dressing intact.
    c. Using sterile gloves, release the dressing on one end, inspect the insertion site, and reattach the dressing.
    d. Palpate the insertion site for tenderness daily and change gauze dressing every 2 to 3 days.

14. A 35-year-old client has undergone a craniotomy for a meningioma at the base of the frontal lobe. The client was moved from ICU to secondary ICU on the first postoperative day and is doing very well, ambulating independently in the hallway but taking pain medication for persistent headache. The physician has discontinued postoperative heparin and prescribed oral steroids to prevent cerebral edema. The patient is a single mother of a 7-year-old child and insists she be discharged on the second postoperative day so she can return home to her child. Which of the other healthcare disciplines should the CNL recommend evaluate the client prior to discharge to determine her readiness?

    a. Psychologist.
    b. Physical therapist.
    c. Occupational therapist.
    d. Social worker.

15. A 19-year-old college student has been hospitalized and diagnosed with stage IIB Hodgkin's disease. The client is refusing all treatments, stating that he is going to use herbal therapy and diet to bring about a cure. He has signed himself out of the hospital and is preparing to leave. The client's nurse is upset and asks the CNL what actions she can take to help ensure the client receives treatment. The CNL advises the nurse that the BEST action is to

    a. Call the client's parents and report his condition.
    b. Tell the client that he is making a terrible mistake that may cost him his life.
    c. Do nothing as the client has a right to refuse treatment.
    d. Provide the client with information about the disease and a list of resources.

16. Three clients in outpatient surgery undergo cholecystectomies but react very differently in the postoperative period.

> One client is awake, asking for food, joking with staff, and wanting to go home.
>
> A second client resists any efforts at interaction and insists he is too weak and uncomfortable to go home.
>
> The third client moans and complains almost continuously about pain, despite pain medications.

This disproportional response is best accounted for by the theory of

    a. Change.
    b. Complexity.
    c. Behavior.
    d. Development.

17. A 65-year-old client is admitted to the unit after 3 days of severe diarrhea and vomiting from gastroenteritis. The client is markedly dehydrated and unable to tolerate oral fluids because of nausea. The physician has left a telephone order for intravenous D5NS for infusion at 300 mL per hour for the initial 2 hours and then 150 mL per hour thereafter. The physician stated she would visit the patient in 2 to 4 hours. The nurse caring for the client is unsure that the IV solution is appropriate and asks the CNL for advice. Which of the following is the BEST advice?

    a. Administer the IV solution as ordered as it is appropriate.
    b. Hold the order until the physician arrives.
    c. Call the physician to clarify the order since the IV solution is hypertonic.
    d. Call the physician to clarify the order since the IV solution is hypotonic.

18. A client with strep throat has had a previous anaphylactic reaction to penicillin, so the physician has ordered cephalexin (250 mg orally every 6 hours). Which of the following should be the CNL's PRIMARY initial concern?

    a. Cephalexin may result in fungal infections.
    b. Cross-hypersensitivity reactions may occur in those with penicillin allergies.
    c. Superinfections may occur with cephalexin.
    d. Cephalexin may result in decreased prothrombin activity.

19. The CNL has instituted the practice of leader rounding and is maintaining a rounding log to keep track of communications with team members. What is the PRIMARY purpose of leader rounding?

    a. Evaluate staff.
    b. Identify problems at an early stage.
    c. Monitor complaints.
    d. Improve relationship between the CNL and team members.

20. A client with end-stage renal disease has been under hospice care for two 90-day periods. His condition has declined, but death is not imminent. The CNL understands that

    a. Hospice care can be extended by unlimited 60-day periods.
    b. Hospice care can be extended by one 60-day period.
    c. Hospice care can be extended by two more 90-day periods.
    d. Hospice care must be discontinued at this time.

The following scenario applies to questions 21 and 22

21. On the pediatric unit, a 3-year-old child with severe nausea and vomiting has been treated with initial boluses of NS for severe dehydration and is now to be maintained on maintenance intravenous fluids. The child weighs 12 kilograms. The physician has ordered dextrose 5% in half-normal saline at the rate of 1,000 mL/day in addition to 50 mL/kg/day for every kilogram above 10 kg of body weight. The CNL anticipates the child will receive how many milliliters (rounded to the nearest whole number) each hour?

a. 42 mL.
b. 46 mL.
c. 92 mL.
d. 83 mL.

22. The IV is to be administered with a microdrip system that has a drop factor of 60 drops/mL. The flow rate per minute at which the IV should be set (rounded to the nearest whole number) to administer the prescribed volume of fluid each hour is

a. 5 drops/min.
b. 50 drops/min.
c. 92 drops/min.
d. 46 drops/min.

23. The CNL is serving on a committee to increase compliance with evidence-based practice guidelines. The hospital's current average door-to-balloon time is 110 minutes. The CNL realizes that the CMS performance target for door-to-balloon time is

a. ≤ 60 minutes.
b. ≤ 90 minutes.
c. ≤ 100 minutes.
d. ≤ 110 minutes.

24. When considering the budget, which costs in a healthcare organization are usually fixed?

a. Surgical supplies.
b. Medical supplies.
c. Administrative salaries.
d. Food costs.

25. Based on research of best practices, the CNL has recommended a number of best practice guidelines to improve patient safety and patient outcomes. Which type of best practice should the CNL generally attempt to institute first?

a. A practice that requires new equipment.
b. A practice that involves the entire staff.
c. A practice that requires organizational change.
d. A practice that requires simple changes in procedure.

26. A client has been admitted to the unit with metastatic ovarian cancer and has chosen to undergo aggressive therapy rather than hospice care. At which point in the client's disease should the CNL recommend that the client receive palliative care?

a. Immediately.
b. After the client completes aggressive therapy.
c. After the client is admitted to hospice care.
d. When the client's pain becomes unmanageable.

27. The CNL is leading a team working with clients who are at-risk for development of heart disease and diabetes because of lifestyle, diet, and obesity. Considering the Health Belief Model, which concept is most likely to affect a person's willingness to make changes?

    a. Perceived severity.
    b. Perceived benefit.
    c. Perceived susceptibility.
    d. Perceived barriers.

28. The CNL's interdisciplinary team is working with a group of males having sex with males (MSM) with a history of sexually transmitted disease. The goal is to promote safe sex practices and prevent reinfection and HIV, providing education, support, and condoms. However, a small subset of the group has been noncompliant. They have sought repeated treatment and some are now HIV positive. Considering Pender's Health Promotion Model, which factor should the CNL consider as most likely influencing this behavior?

    a. Perceived barriers to action.
    b. Activity-related affect.
    c. Interpersonal influences.
    d. Situational influences.

29. The CNL wants to utilize de Bono's Six Thinking Hats technique for thinking and problem solving. With this model, if the CNL functions as the Blue Hat, which of the following actions is the CNL responsible for?

    a. Providing objective facts and figures.
    b. Discussing negative and positive feelings and responses.
    c. Serving as devil's advocate.
    d. Facilitating the discussion and providing structure.

30. Which of the following is an example of using a normative re-educative strategy to facilitate and manage change?

    a. The CNL encourages the team to identify problems and solutions.
    b. The CNL provides facts and figures gleaned from research to support change.
    c. The CNL uses authority to demand that staff make changes.
    d. The CNL utilizes a method of rewards and punishment to promote change.

31. The CNL has identified a number of changes to promote safety and improve client outcomes and has the support of most members of the interdisciplinary team in working toward change. However, two members of the team remain vocally resistant to change and are arguing with other team members, trying to convince them to resist changes as well. The BEST solution for the CNL is to

    a. Ignore the two team members.
    b. Ask to have the two team members transferred to a different unit.
    c. Tell the two team members that they are being disruptive.
    d. Ask the two team members to take active roles in facilitating change.

32. A CNL is from a low-context culture (the United States) but works on a team with a number of immigrant staff from high-context cultures (Japan, Mexico, Fiji, Saudi Arabia). The CNL expects that the biggest disparity between the CNL and the team members will be with

    a. Communication style.
    b. Cognitive ability.
    c. Ethical standards.
    d. Work ethic.

33. Which of the following is the safest method for physicians to order medications?

    a. Handwritten order.
    b. Verbal order.
    c. Telephone order.
    d. Computerized physician order entry.

34. The CNL is a new graduate and part of the Millennial generation but is working with an interdisciplinary team comprised primarily of Baby Boomers and Generation Xers. Considering generational differences, the CNL is probably

    a. More comfortable with new technology.
    b. More likely to be skeptical of traditional practices.
    c. More like to have respect for authority.
    d. More likely to question authority.

35. The CNL gives a presentation to the board of directors outlining the cost-effectiveness of the CNL's role, utilizing organizational data that shows reduction in infections and patient injuries. This is primarily an example of

    a. Self-promotion.
    b. Staff education.
    c. Professional advocacy.
    d. Research.

36. Which of the following is an example of an indirect patient care function of the CNL?

    a. Patient education.
    b. Coordination of care.
    c. Communication.
    d. Leadership.

37. In the event of a disaster, which initial strategy could be employed to increase a hospital's surge capacity?

    a. Identify clients safely eligible for early discharge.
    b. Place extra beds in private rooms.
    c. Recommend closing the emergency department to nondisaster-related clients.
    d. Transfer clients so that open rooms are in close proximity.

38. Which of the following is part of the suprasystem of a hospital?

    a. A self-contained research facility.
    b. A laboratory.
    c. An accrediting agency.
    d. Security.

39. The CNL is utilizing the STAR model to facilitate systems change. According to this model, a change in one area usually

    a. Is unsuccessful.
    b. Results in unsuspected outcomes.
    c. Promotes acceptance of change.
    d. Necessitates change in another.

40. According to Systems Theory (Bertalanffy), if *input* comprises the team members and clients and *throughput* comprises the CNL's supervision and management of nursing care the clients receive, which of the following is an expected *output*?

    a. Improved staff satisfaction.
    b. Improved client care and outcomes.
    c. Identification of problems.
    d. Increased accountability.

41. According to the CNL Standards of Conduct, concern for and advocating for the welfare of clients and staff and demonstrating understanding of others' beliefs and values is related to

    a. Accountability.
    b. Altruism.
    c. Integrity
    d. Social justice.

42. Which is the BEST way to communicate changes in processes to team members?

    a. Make an announcement during team meetings.
    b. Tell each staff person individually.
    c. Post a memo on a communication board.
    d. Utilize multiple and repeated means of communication.

43. The CNL utilizes a communication board to provide information to team members. How frequently should the CNL plan to update the communication board?

    a. Quarterly.
    b. Monthly.
    c. Weekly.
    d. Daily.

44. When the CNL plans to initiate a change in processes or procedures, which is the MOST important factor to communicate to staff?

    a. Reason.
    b. Cost effectiveness.
    c. Timeframe.
    d. Learning curve.

45. The PRIMARY purpose of the client rounding log is to

    a. Ensure nurses are seeing clients on a regularly scheduled basis.
    b. Improve client outcomes.
    c. Monitor individual staff.
    d. Prevent client neglect.

46. The CNL receives complaints from two clients and one team member that another member of the team has been acting in a grossly inappropriate and unprofessional manner, but the CNL has not observed this behavior. Which of the following initial actions is MOST appropriate?

- a. Consult with human resources.
- b. Conduct interviews with the clients and reporting team member to gain more information.
- c. Confront the accused team member with the allegations.
- d. Observe the accused team member closely for a number of days before making a decision about action.

47. A team member approached the CNL and reported that he felt there was "something wrong" with a client even though the client's vital signs seemed stable, and the client had no specific complaints but appeared slightly restless. Subsequently, the client experienced sudden onset of chest pain and shortness of breath. What type of thinking was the nurse exhibiting?

- a. Critical.
- b. Reflective.
- c. Problem-solving.
- d. Intuitive.

48. The CNL is using the DESK model to counsel a team member who needs to improve performance. Which action does the CNL carry out first?

- a. Delineating steps the staff person must take.
- b. Describing the problem behavior.
- c. Defending the CNL's need to take action.
- d. Describing punitive actions if the staff person fails to improve.

49. Which ratio of recognition to criticism is most effective in maintaining a positive culture?

- a. 1:1.
- b. 1:2.
- c. 3:1.
- d. 2:1.

50. The CNL is interviewing nurses for a position on the team, using a behavioral interview technique and the EAR model to record the interviewees' answers. Therefore, the CNL is recording information about the

- a. Event, action, and results.
- b. Education, adaptation, and reaction.
- c. Encounter, agreement, and recall.
- d. Evidence, action, and recommendation.

51. The CNL must hire a new nursing team member and has conducted the initial interviews and will send three candidates to a peer interview with other team members. The final decision about hiring will rest with the team members. Because of this, the most important factor in making a selection of three candidates is

    a. The CNL choses candidates who are similar to those already on the team.

    b. The CNL choses those with the best qualifications.

    c. The CNL choses a candidate who seems excellent and two candidates that seem weak to ensure the preferred candidate will be hired.

    d. The CNL would be willing to hire any of the three selected candidates.

52. Which of the following questions may a CNL LEGALLY ask an applicant for a position on the team?

    a. "When did you graduate from nursing school?"

    b. "Would you have a problem working a 12-hour shift?"

    c. "Do you have any disabilities that may affect your work?"

    d. "How long have you lived in this area?"

53. The CNL has a newly hired team member and believes that mentoring is the best approach to ensure that the team member is well trained and understands the needs of the position. Which of the following is the BEST approach?

    a. The CNL serves as the mentor.

    b. The CNL asks a high-performing team member to serve as mentor.

    c. The CNL asks the newly hired team member if he or she would like to have a mentor.

    d. The CNL suggests the newly hired team member choose a mentor from the team.

54. When applying the nursing process to the process of education when providing training for team members on health promotion strategies, what does the CNL do as part of implementation?

    a. Develop teaching plan.

    b. Assess learning needs.

    c. Evaluate outcomes.

    d. Carry out instruction.

55. When the CNL is working on quality improvement, which type of chart may be most helpful to present a schematic representation of a process?

    a. Flow chart.

    b. Pareto chart.

    c. Control chart.

    d. Run chart.

56. The CNL is conducting leader rounds, visiting with each client on the medical-surgical unit, and finds that 6 of 30 clients report having to use the call bell to ask for pain medication in the previous 24 hours. Based on this finding, the CNL believes that

    a. Care related to pain management is adequate.

    b. Care related to pain management is inadequate.

    c. Care has been negligent.

    d. Staffing is probably inadequate.

57. The CNL in an outpatient surgical unit notes an increasing number of no-shows and late arrivals for surgical procedures, resulting in lost revenue and added costs, as staff often have to work late. Which initial intervention is likely to be most effective?

    a. Ask the physicians to remind clients to arrive on time.
    b. Send reminders to patient by mail.
    c. Make pre-visit telephone calls a day or two prior to surgery.
    d. Schedule procedures later in the day.

58. The CNL plans to institute hourly nursing rounds for all clients on the unit, and the team members are questioning how they will know there is benefit to the procedure. Which of the following is most likely to convince the staff of the value of hourly rounds?

    a. Conduct a pre- and post-evaluation of the average number of call bells over a specified time period.
    b. Provide staff with evidence-based research from institutions that utilize hourly rounds.
    c. Conduct patient satisfaction surveys.
    d. Conduct staff satisfaction surveys.

59. Which of the following poses the greatest risk to an organization's computer network security?

    a. Spyware.
    b. Shoulder surfing.
    c. Removable storage devices.
    d. Malicious insiders.

60. The hospital has collected data regarding patient falls resulting in no injury and patient falls resulting in injury. How should the information be differentiated in order to utilize the information most effectively for quality improvement?

    a. By organization.
    b. By discipline.
    c. By unit.
    d. By individual staff.

61. Which of the following is the most efficient method of reminding staff members to educate clients about the need for vaccinations?

    a. Remind staff during a staff meeting.
    b. Imbed prompts in the clinical information system/electronic health record.
    c. Post reminders on a communication board.
    d. Place posters about immunizations in prominent areas about the unit.

62 The primary difference between a data warehouse and a data mart is that

    a. The data warehouse is a smaller component of the larger data mart.
    b. The data mart is a smaller component of the larger data warehouse.
    c. There is no difference as the terms are interchangeable.
    d. The data mart is not accessible to data mining.

63. The CNL has instituted the use of the Situation-Background-Assessment-Recommendation (SBAR) communication technique to facilitate communication among healthcare providers about clients. With this technique, which of the following information should be provided as part of Background?

    a. Patient's name and diagnosis.
    b. Review of plan of care.
    c. Current vital signs and description of pain.
    d. Review all tubes, lines, and drains.

64. The BEST initial question to ask a client when utilizing individualized patient care (IPC) is

    a. "What three things can we do to make sure you receive excellent care?"
    b. "What do you expect of your nurses?"
    c. "How can I help you?"
    d. "Do you have any questions?"

65. When using the AIDET technique (acknowledge, introduce, duration, explanation, thanks) when treating a client, an appropriate first statement is

    a. "I need to take your blood pressure."
    b. "Good afternoon, I'm going to take your blood pressure."
    c. "Hello, this will only take a minute."
    d. "Good afternoon, Mrs. Smith."

66. In a service recovery model, the first step of the CNL is usually to

    a. Avoid acknowledging blame.
    b. Acknowledge the problem and apologize.
    c. Attempt to correct the situation.
    d. Determine the cause of the problem.

67. A client asks for the CNL and begins angrily denouncing his primary care nurse as incompetent, shouting at the CNL, and throwing his call bell onto the floor. What is the BEST response?

    a. "I cannot talk to you until you calm down."
    b. "Your nurse is very capable."
    c. "Your behavior is unacceptable."
    d. "I would like to help you, but first I need to understand what the problem is."

68. The CNL has analyzed data regarding infection rates, falls, and client satisfaction, and believes that the unit requires the addition of another nurse in order to improve client care and client satisfaction. When approaching the senior management to request another position, the best approach is generally to focus on

    a. Cost-effectiveness.
    b. Improved client care.
    c. Client satisfaction.
    d. Staff needs.

69. Which of the following is an example of "cost shifting"?

a. The hospital decreases costs of care in the ED because of increased traffic.
b. The hospital moves expenses from one budget category to another.
c. The hospital increases ED costs to private pay and insured clients to offset loss from those with no insurance.
d. The hospital changes costs on a monthly basis, reflecting income.

70. The CNL notes when making rounds that team members are leaving extra linen (towels, sheets, washcloths) in the clients' private rooms in case they are needed later. During the team meeting, the CNL notes that

a. This is a good time-saving practice.
b. This is not a cost-effective practice.
c. This increases the risk of contamination.
d. This is a violation of health practices.

71. The CNL's team comprises the following (per week):

CNL: 40 hours.
6 RNs: 40 hours each.
4 RNs: 20 hours each.
2 LVNs: 40 hours each.

Based on the above figures, how many nursing FTEs are employed each week?

a. 13.
b. 12.
c. 11.
d. 10.

72. The CNL is calculating worked hours per patient day (WHPPD) and has budgeted 8 WHPPD, so nurses are expected to provide 8 hours of direct client care in 24 hours. However, nurses required 10 hours to deliver direct client care. What percentage of productivity is the unit operating at?

a. 8%
b. 125%
c. 12.5%
d. 80%

73. When looking at benchmarks, the CNL notes that the unit ranks 69% in one category. This means that the unit

a. Scored higher than 69% of those benchmarked against.
b. Scored lower than 69% of those benchmarked against.
c. Has an actual score of 31%.
d. Scored higher than 31% of those benchmarked against.

74. On the Hospital Consumer Assessment of Healthcare Providers and Systems (HCAPHS) survey, one question asks how often nurses carefully listened to the client. The hospital scored as follows:

72% Always.
18% Usually.
8% Sometimes.
2% Never.

Which score will be reported on *Hospital Compare?*

a. All scores.
b. 90%
c. 2%.
d. 72%.

75. The CNL reviews the patient satisfaction survey scores for the ED and finds that the department has consistently scored low on promptly responding to requests for information despite repeated discussions about keeping clients informed. Which of the following steps should the CNL undertake first?

a. Ask for assistance from human resources.
b. Show the staff the results and asks the reason for poor results.
c. Filter the surveys by shift.
d. Establish a reward system for improved scores.

76. In the nominal group technique, the CNL as group leader identifies an issue, and then the FIRST step to decision-making is

a. Team members discuss the ideas.
b. Team members present their ideas to the group.
c. Team members write out ideas without discussion.
d. Team members vote.

77. The primary advantage of the Delphi decision-making technique is that

a. Group members don't need to meet face to face.
b. Group meetings are streamlined.
c. Extensive discussion takes place.
d. It is especially suitable for small groups.

78. The CNL is using the PLEASED technique to evaluate information gleaned from the Internet:

P: Purpose.
L: Links
E: Editorial.
A. Author.
S: Site navigation.
E: Ethical disclosures.
D: ?

What does the D in the mnemonic stand for?

a. Data.
b. Description.
c. Discussion
d. Date of last update.

The following scenario applies to questions 79 and 80

A 78-year-old client who has undergone a hip replacement is in the first postoperative day and has been recovering well, but when the nurse does an hourly round, she finds the client exhibiting sudden onset of acute change in mental status. He is agitated and disoriented, and his speech is rambling at times, but symptoms are fluctuating.

79. When discussing the assessment with the nurse, the CNL suggest that the nurse administer the

a. Mini-Cog exam.
b. Mini-Mental State Exam (MMSE).
c. Palliative Performance Scale.
d. Confusion Assessment Method.

80. Based on the client's symptom profile and probable diagnosis, the CNL anticipates that the physician will order which medication to relieve symptoms?

a. Morphine sulfate.
b. Paroxetine.
c. Lorazepam.
d. Gabapentin.

81. The CNL is assuming leadership of a team comprised of staff members who have been working in the same or similar positions for 3 to 5 years. Based on Benner's model of novice to expert, the CNL should anticipate that most members would be classified as

a. Advanced beginners.
b. Competent.
c. Proficient.
d. Novice.

82. The CNL encourages team members to gain leadership experience. One novice team member states she doesn't understand the need to develop leadership skills since she is not part of management and has little experience. Which of the following is the best response?

a. "Everyone needs leadership experience."
b. "Leadership skills will help you be more effective when working with clients, other nurses, and unlicensed assistive personnel."
c. "If you want to advance, you need leadership skills."
d. "While you may not see the value of leadership skills now, you will understand the value as you gain experience."

83. The CNL had been very successful in one leadership position using a democratic style of leadership and believes this is the best leadership approach. However, he has encountered resistance in a new position and has received poor ratings from peers. Which of the following theories may help the CNL understand this disparity?

a. Contingency theory.
b. Change theory.
c. Institutional theory.
d. Management theory.

84. The CNL and his team have developed a successful strategy to ensure discharge instructions are effectively reviewed with clients. Utilizing horizontal leadership, the CNL would expect to provide this information to other teams by

    a. Sending data to the unit supervisor to review and disseminate.
    b. Sharing directly with other teams.
    c. Sending data to the chief nursing officer to review and disseminate.
    d. Asking the certified nurse educator to review data and disseminate results.

85. When working on strategies for disease prevention, the CNL recognizes that the ethnic group with the lowest life expectancy in the United States is

    a. African Americans.
    b. Native Americans.
    c. Hispanics.
    d. Pacific Islanders.

86. The CNL is utilizing Juran's quality improvement process to facilitate change. Which of the following should the CNL do initially?

    a. List problems and prioritize them.
    b. Conduct root-cause analysis.
    c. Consider various alternative solutions.
    d. Monitor control system.

87. The CNL's team utilizes the "Five Whys" method to help determine cause and solve problems. An elderly client who recently had a hip replacement climbed over the bedrails and fell, resulting in the need for a return to surgery to repair the hip. Utilizing the "Five Whys" method, which of the following should be the first question?

    a. "Why did the client fall?"
    b. "Why did the client climb over the bedrails?"
    c. "What could have prevented the client climbing over the bedrails?"
    d. "What action should the team take to prevent this from happening in the future?"

88. The CNL's team has focused on teaching hospitalized chronic asthma and COPD patients to monitor their health and control symptoms, using individual protocols for treatment. Which type of data collection is most indicated to measure outcomes?

    a. Client surveys (paper).
    b. Client telephone interviews.
    c. Readmission data.
    d. Observation of clients.

89. The CNL wants to collect data about patient satisfaction with outpatient treatment. Which of the following may be utilized for quantitative data collection?

    a. In-depth open-ended interviews.
    b. Interviews asking each participant the exact same questions.
    c. Observation.
    d. Serial open-ended interviews.

90. Which of the following is an example of a provider-focused outcome?

    a. Pain control.
    b. Client satisfaction.
    c. Hospital-wide mortality rates.
    d. Nurse turnover.

91. The CNL leads a team on the substance abuse rehabilitation unit and is involved in a community partnership, working with adolescents and trying to overcome predictive/risk factors and reinforce protective factors. Which of the following is a protective factor for substance abuse for an adolescent whose parents are drug abusers?

    a. Knowledge about the risks of substance abuse.
    b. Uncertainty about future plans.
    c. Poor reading and academic skills.
    d. Early sexual activity.

92. The CNL is analyzing conflict in the workplace and finds that two nurses have exhibited persistent conflict. When the CNL talks with the nurses, it is clear that they have no trust in each other, and this impairs their ability to work together. Which type of factor is the cause of this conflict?

    a. Professional difference.
    b. Organizational factor.
    c. Individual characteristic.
    d. Interpersonal factor.

93. Two members of the team, a proficient nurse and a novice nurse, come separately to the CNL and state they want to quit the team and transfer to another unit because they cannot work together. The first nurse tries to avoid all conflict, but the novice nurse is more confrontational. During a recent disagreement, the proficient nurse tried to leave the situation, but the novice nurse followed her, arguing and making the proficient nurse feel threatened. The proficient nurse pushed the novice nurse away, causing the novice nurse to feel attacked. What appears to be the primary cause of the conflict?

    a. Differences in professional experience.
    b. Differences in values.
    c. Differences in communication strategies.
    d. Differences in work ethics.

94. Which analytical method is used to compare the average cost of an event (such as a stage IV pressure sores) and the cost of intervention (such as additional staff and better wound treatment) to demonstrate savings?

    a. Cost-benefit analysis.
    b. Cost-effective analysis.
    c. Cost-utility analysis.
    d. Efficacy study.

95. Hospital A is near a number of large retirement communities, so budgeting for anticipated revenue is based on a payor mix that averages 68% Medicare patients, 10% Medicaid patients, 8% insurance, 5% self-pay, 5% HMO/PPO, and 4% uninsured. Hospital B is of equal size and is 25 miles away, It has a payor mix of 45% Medicare patients, 36% insurance, 9% HMO/PPO, 5% Medicaid,4% self-pay, and 1% uninsured. Based on this information, which hospital is likely to receive the most reimbursement for services?

    a. Hospital A.
    b. Hospital B.
    c. Reimbursement should be about the same.
    d. Reimbursement cannot be predicted.

96. The CNL is developing strategies to decrease the incidence of catheter-associated urinary tract infections by eliminating the use of indwelling urinary catheters unless absolutely necessary. Considering current CDC recommendations, which of the following clients should the CNL recommend NOT receive an indwelling catheter?

    a. A 72-year-old patient with a stage III sacral pressure sore.
    b. A 66-year-old patient with bladder outlet obstruction.
    c. An 82-year-old patient with chronic urinary incontinence.
    d. A 52-year-old patient critically ill with heart failure.

97. Which type of operational budget requires that each cost center have revenue and costs determined for the entire budget period and a fixed budget developed?

    a. Zero-based.
    b. Forecast.
    c. Rolling.
    d. Flexible.

98. The CNL's *span of control* refers to

    a. The unit to which a CNL is responsible.
    b. The number of disciplines that report to the CNL.
    c. The functions for which the CNL is responsible.
    d. The number of staff persons who report to the CNL.

99. As part of shared governance, the CNL serves on the clinical practice partnership council. What is usually the primary purpose of a clinical practice council?

    a. Make recommendations related to hiring and promotions.
    b. Establish nursing practice standards.
    c. Ensure nursing standards are upheld.
    d. Assess the educational needs of the staff and implement educational programs.

100. SWOT analysis is most commonly used to develop a(n)

    a. Strategic plan for an organization.
    b. Plan of care.
    c. Operating budget.
    d. Education plan.

101. The CNL asks the team to brainstorm a problem during a meeting and come up with a number of possible solutions to discuss. This type of exercise is an example of

- a. Convergent thinking.
- b. Divergent thinking.
- c. Critical thinking.
- d. Divergent thinking.

102. Which of the following would be considered grounds for sanctions against the CNL by the Commission on Nurse Certification?

- a. The CNL is convicted of a misdemeanor traffic violation.
- b. The CNL is fired without cause during his probationary period.
- c. The CNL confused two clients with similar names and administered treatment to the wrong client.
- d. The CNL is found to be grossly negligent in caring for a client.

103. The primary concern of risk management in healthcare today is

- a. Prevention of financial loss.
- b. Patient safety.
- c. Education.
- d. Defense of malpractice claims.

104. The CNL in the intensive care unit notes when evaluating the unit that the rate of central line–associated infections is higher than in other hospital units and higher than benchmarks. What should the CNL recommend as the next action?

- a. Provide education to ICU staff.
- b. Reprimand ICU staff.
- c. Conduct root-cause analysis.
- d. Ask risk management to assess financial liabilities.

105. The CNL notes that one team leader on her unit is very autocratic and asks for little input from her team members. The team leader is an excellent nurse and is very well organized, but team members resent her, and turnover on her team is high. Which of the following actions by the CNL is most likely to be productive?

- a. Reprimand the team leader.
- b. Help the team leader develop an action plan to improve leadership skills.
- c. Outline the team leader's leadership failings.
- d. Advise the team members to express their concerns to the team leader.

106. The hospital that the CNL is employed at is applying for Magnet status. What type of management style is required of those institutions that receive Magnet recognition?

- a. Participative/Collaborative.
- b. Democratic.
- c. Consultative
- d. Autocratic.

107. In states (such as California) or organizations that mandate a specific patient to nurse ratio, under what circumstances may the patient to nurse ratio generally be bypassed?

    a. None.
    b. Staff absenteeism.
    c. Financial constraints.
    d. Health emergencies.

108. When calculating nurse to patient ratios, which of the following are generally included?

    a. All licensed nurses and unlicensed assistive personnel involved in direct patient care.
    b. All licensed nurses and nurse managers.
    c. All licensed nurses involved in direct client care.
    d. All licensed nurses and unlicensed assistive personnel and all nurse managers.

109. The CNL is preparing a professional resume. Which of the following should the CNL avoid?

    a. Bolding.
    b. Plain type font.
    c. Two-column format.
    d. Key words.

110. Which of the following is the primary measure of quality practice for a CNL?

    a. Improved clinical/cost outcomes.
    b. Staff satisfaction.
    c. Client satisfaction.
    d. Nursing hours per patient day.

111. The CNL should base clinical practice guidelines on

    a. Experience.
    b. Evidence.
    c. Expert advice.
    d. Common practice.

112. The CNL on a geriatric unit observes that a recently graduated nurse appears uncomfortable with family members of dying clients and avoids talking or interacting with them when providing patient care. When a client's daughter began crying while the nurse was turning the client, the nurse didn't look at or speak to the daughter but abruptly left the room. Which is the BEST approach for the CNL to take?

    a. Reassign the nurse to clients who are not dying.
    b. Describe the incident to the nurse and ask for an explanation.
    c. Give the nurse literature about death and dying.
    d. Practice role-playing with the nurse.

113. What is the most important factor in ensuring clients participate fully in care?

    a. Age.
    b. Learning style.
    c. Health literacy.
    d. Motivation.

114. The CNL anticipates that in the future Medicare payments will be increasingly

a. Performance-based.
b. Reduced.
c. Standardized on a national basis.
d. Fee-for-service based.

The following scenario applies to questions 115 and 116

A client was admitted to an acute care hospital under the Medicare Inpatient Prospective Payment System (IPPS). When documenting diagnoses that were present on admission (POA), the nurse failed to examine the client's sacral area to observe for a pressure sore. However, a small sacral pressure sore was documented 2 days after admission when noted by an unlicensed assistive personnel who was bathing the client. Subsequently, the pressure sore enlarged and required debridement and prolonged treatment. The pressure sore was noted and coded on discharge papers.

115. When considering reimbursement for the condition, the CNL anticipates that Medicare

a. Will pay for the condition.
b. Will not pay for the condition.
c. Will require the POA diagnoses be corrected before payment is issued.
d. Will fine the hospital.

116. Because of this nurse's oversight, the initial action of the CNL should be to

a. Reprimand the nurse.
b. Remind team members of the importance of examining clients for pressure sores.
c. Review admission procedures and admission forms.
d. Require all team members to review admission procedures.

117. It is the CNL's responsibility to ensure that staff members in ambulatory care are meeting National Patient Safety Goals. Under the Joint Commission's Ambulatory Care National Patient Safety Goals (2014), the three steps that healthcare providers must take to prevent mistakes in surgery are (1) ensure surgery is on the correct patient and correct body part, (2) mark the correct place on the patient's body, and (3)

a. Use proven guidelines to prevent infection.
b. Pause before surgery to ensure mistakes aren't being made.
c. Complete a pre-surgical checklist.
d. Utilize the most current surgical technique.

118. While patient safety has improved, the CNL observes that injuries to nursing staff and unlicensed assistive personnel on the medical-surgical unit have increased, resulting in increased absenteeism and increased costs to the unit. The CNL notes that most injuries occur when staff members are lifting or transferring patients, especially because many patients are overweight. Which is the BEST solution to the problem?

a. Establish a comprehensive safe patient-handling program.
b. Warn staff members to get help with lifting and transferring patients.
c. Flag the rooms of overweight patients so staff knows to get assistance.
d. Place posters that demonstrate safe lifting around the unit.

119. The two elements that are essential for a nurse and patient to establish a therapeutic alliance are

- a. Trust and positivity.
- b. Knowledge and competence.
- c. Time and patience.
- d. Mutuality and reciprocity.

120. When a patient is admitted to the orthopedic unit with a fractured femur, the intake assessment includes not only questions about the orthopedic problem but also questions about social history, family history, nutrition, habits and lifestyle, sexuality, spirituality, and health concerns. This is an example of a(n)

- a. Holistic assessment.
- b. Problem-focused assessment.
- c. Emergency assessment.
- d. Ongoing assessment.

121. The epidemiological triad comprises

- a. Data, surveillance, and analysis.
- b. Agent, vector, and host.
- c. Agent, host, and environment.
- d. Data, analysis, and outcomes.

122. When accessing information regarding best practices, which of the following resources would be considered the most valid?

- a. Journal article (juried).
- b. WebMD (Internet site).
- c. *60 Minutes* (CBS TV program).
- d. Dr. Oz (cardiothoracic surgeon and TV personality)

123. STOPP and START criteria are utilized to prevent

- a. Falls and client injuries.
- b. Medication interactions and incorrect prescriptions.
- c. Transfusion reactions.
- d. Surgical errors.

124. A 76-year-old client has fallen three times in the past month. The CNL reviews the client's list of medications to determine whether the falls are related to medications.

> Diphenhydramine (Benadryl) 50 mg twice daily for allergies.
> Metoprolol 50 mg twice daily for supraventricular tachycardia and hypertension.
> Bupropion (Wellbutrin) sustained release 150 mg/day for mild depression.
> PEG solution (Miralax) 1 package in 8 ounces of water as needed for constipation.
> Levothyroxine (Synthroid) 112 mcg daily.

Which of the medications is most likely a cause for concern in an older adult?

- a. Metoprolol.
- b. Bupropion.
- c. Levothyroxine.
- d. Diphenhydramine.

125. The CNL works in a well-baby clinic and is planning educational programs for parents of toddlers. Which of the following topic would be of MOST value to a group of parents with children ranging from 1 to 3 years of age?

    a. SIDS.
    b. Child abuse.
    c. Preventing injuries.
    d. Common childhood illnesses.

126. A nurse on the CNL's team states she is unsure how to assess cyanosis in a very dark-skinned individual. The CNL advises the nurse to inspect the client's

    a. Nail beds.
    b. Conjunctiva.
    c. Fingers.
    d. Toes.

127. A 24-year-old client's father has been diagnosed with Huntington disease, an autosomal dominantly inherited disease. Which of the following statements by the client suggests a need for further education about the disease?

    a. "I may be a carrier even if I don't have the disease."
    b. "There's a 50% chance I may have the disease."
    c. "Only one parent needs to pass on a defective gene."
    d. "I can wait to be tested since there is no effective treatment."

128. A homeless client is to be discharged after hospitalization for diagnosis and treatment of tuberculosis, but the client must continue to take medication regularly. The client lives under a freeway overpass and resists efforts to house him but goes every day for lunch at the Salvation Army. Which of the following should the CNL advise as the BEST approach to ensure that the client complete the medication regimen?

    a. Provide the client with all of the medications needed for a full course of treatment.
    b. Arrange for directly observed treatment (DOT) at the Salvation Army.
    c. Arrange for transportation to bring the client to the hospital for treatment.
    d. Get a court order to force the client into a supervised housing situation where medication can be administered.

129. The CNL is utilizing the 8Ps of Risk Assessment to identify older adult clients at risk after discharge from an inpatient facility: Problem medications, Psychological, Principal diagnosis, Polypharmacy, Poor health literacy, Patient support, Prior hospitalization, and Palliative care. Which of the following is the primary concern when assessing the "Psychological" category?

    a. Bipolar disorder.
    b. Neuroses.
    c. Personality disorders.
    d. Depression or history of depression.

130. In the area of public policy, three players comprise the "iron triangle" because of the extent of their control of policy development. These 3 players are (1) the executive agency responsible for a policy area, (2) Congress and Congressional committees and subcommittees, and (3)

 a. Corporations.
 b. General public.
 c. Interest groups/Lobbyists.
 d. State legislatures.

131. According to Kingdon's Model of Policy Formulation (2003), which of the following is required before a problem is placed on the agenda in the problem stream?

 a. Financial support.
 b. A possible solution.
 c. Timeframe for solution.
 d. Public support.

132. The CNL serves on a committee lobbying the state legislature to enact nurse-patient ratios. Which of the following current issues in nursing may work against enacting ratios?

 a. Nursing shortage.
 b. Nursing salaries.
 c. Nursing education.
 d. Nursing processes.

133. A CNL is employed in a behavioral health organization. Recently, a client was discharged after 6 weeks of inpatient therapy and committed suicide within 24 hours of discharge. What action does the CNL anticipate that the Joint Commission will require of the organization?

 a. No action as the client committed suicide after discharge.
 b. Disciplinary action against discharging physician.
 c. Notification of the Joint Commission.
 d. Root cause analysis.

134. The CNL oversees client care that is provided by a number of different disciplines, (physicians, nurses, social workers, rehabilitation therapists, occupational therapists, physical therapists) and provided in different settings (hospital, clinic, long-term care facility) throughout the continuum of care from admission to post-discharge The CNL takes an active role in assessing and communicating client needs, ensuring that all are working together effectively and meeting the needs of the client. This is an example of

 a. Vertical leadership.
 b. Horizontal leadership.
 c. Lateral integration.
 d. Case management.

135. The parents of a terminally ill 15-year-old client decided to continue aggressive treatments that might extend the client's life for a short period but not bring about a cure. However, the client is adamant about wanting treatment discontinued and begging the staff to help him "die in peace." The physician and nursing staff are conflicted about the parents' decision, but the physician states he must abide by the parents' wishes. Which of the following is the BEST response by the CNL?

- a. Ask the ethics committee for guidance.
- b. Tell the client that his parents have the right to decide.
- c. Ask the parents to reconsider their decision.
- d. Ask the administration to seek a court order requiring discontinuation of treatment.

136. According to Kohlberg's moral development process (1971), what should one expect of a person at the Conventional Level?

- a. Person determines whether something is good or bad depending on consequences.
- b. Person understands personal responsibilities and societal expectations.
- c. Person wants approval from others.
- d. Person does not understand underlying moral codes.

137. According to the American Hospital Association's Patient Care Partnership document, clients should expect

- a. Fair pricing.
- b. Respect for values and spiritual beliefs.
- c. Immediate response to needs.
- d. Management of pain.

138. A team member tells the CNL that when asking a client to sign a surgery permission document, the client stated that the physician had not discussed surgical options or possible complications with the client. The team member also noted that the client seemed confused about the scheduled procedure. What is the BEST action for the CNL?

- a. Report the physician to the ethics committee.
- b. Ask the nurse to call the physician and report the observations.
- c. Call the physician and report the team member's observations.
- d. Provide the client with information about the procedure.

139. The primary responsibility of an ethics committee is to

- a. Provide guidance.
- b. Make decisions.
- c. Conduct risk management.
- d. Provide resources

140. If the WHO and CDC have issued a notice of the alert phase of an influenza pandemic, which of the following actions does the CNL anticipate needs to be carried out at a local and national level?

- a. Stockpiling of drugs.
- b. Isolation procedures.
- c. Establishment of emergency facilities.
- d. Risk assessment.

141. The CNL is considering applying to four different hospitals, but they have different organizational forms. Which of the following organizational forms is likely to present the most challenges in facilitating client-centered, interdisciplinary care?

    a. Program.
    b. Matrix.
    c. Functional.
    d. Parallel.

142. The CNL has made a decision about nursing processes and is aware that there will be resistance from some staff members even though the CNL believes the decision will improve client outcomes based on evidence-based research. Which of the following is the BEST solution?

    a. Ask for input about the issue to make the staff members feel they have a say but carry out the original plans.
    b. Announce the decision, providing evidence-based rationale and establishing evaluation procedures.
    c. Ask for input and allow staff members to vote on whether they want the changes or not.
    d. Announce the decision, informing staff members they must comply.

The following scenario applies to questions 143 and 144

> The CNL is reviewing a proposed purchase of new equipment and is making a report to the board about the expected return on investment (ROI). The following expenses are outlined:
>
> Yearly cost for employees utilizing equipment: $100,000
>
> Percentage of time (in decimals) employees will use equipment: 25% = 0.25
>
> Percentage of estimated increased efficiency (in decimals): 25% = 0.25
>
> Equipment/training costs: $50,000

143. Based on these figures, what are the productivity costs in dollars (excluding costs for depreciation and upgrades)?

    a. $62,500
    b. $50,000
    c. $25,000
    d. $6,250

144. How many months will be required for the equipment to pay for itself?

    a. 8 months.
    b. 25 months.
    c. 48 months.
    d. 96 months.

145. The CNL is working in a disease management (DM) program. Which component of the program must be carried out first?

a. Population identification processes.
b. Evidence-based practice guidelines.
c. Client education for self-management.
d. Evaluation/Outcomes measurement processes.

146. The acute care setting where the CNL is employed utilizes the Patient Intensity for Nursing Index (PINI) system. The four dimensions of nursing intensity include (1) illness severity, (2) dependency on nursing care, (3) complexity of condition, and (4)

a. Resources needed to provide care.
b. Equipment needed to provide care.
c. Time necessary to provide care.
d. Staff needed to provide care.

147. The CNL works on an orthopedic unit with a wide range of clients and is analyzing raw data to determine whether a change in nurse-client ratios has decreased hospital stay. Which of the following is the MOST important to ensure the interpretation is valid?

a. Risk adjustment.
b. Computer-generated data.
c. Number of data elements.
d. Time period.

148. A transformational leader

a. Transforms work processes.
b. Changes personal methods of leadership.
c. Relies on others to take leadership roles.
d. Makes team members feel important and value their work.

149. The CNL is newly hired for a position on a medical-surgical unit in order to improve client outcomes and staff retention because a number of medical errors have occurred and staff turnover is high. Clients have been assigned to nurses by number, with each nurse responsible for the same number of clients, but staff members frequently complain about the inequity of work load. More experienced nurses are usually assigned the most time-intensive clients. Which of the following actions is MOST likely to be effective?

a. Change to a client-acuity staffing pattern.
b. Assign more unlicensed assistive personnel to assist those with time-intensive clients.
c. Assign time-intensive clients more equitably.
d. Leave one nurse unassigned so that person can assist other nurses as needed.

150. One member of the team refuses to acknowledge that there is any conflict among the team members and states he prefers to leave well enough alone. Which strategy for conflict resolution is the team member utilizing?

a. Avoiding.
b. Smoothing over/Reassuring.
c. Withholding/Withdrawing.
d. Accommodating.

Answer Key and Explanations

1. A: The most critical element in the selection of an electronic medical record system is completion of a needs assessment. Most vendors offer different packages and EMRs with different capabilities. Different units of the hospital may have different needs, so the EMR may need to be customizable. For example, the EMRs for pediatrics may need to be set up to evaluate growth and to provide information about childhood immunizations, while the EMR for the emergency department may have quite different needs.

2. D: Ethical decision-making begins with gathering data to determine the issues and the facts as well as to identify moral conflicts. This is followed by identifying key participants and their power to make decisions, level of competence, and rights. Then, one must determine the moral perspective of the participants and phase of moral development before determining desired outcomes and identifying options. Once a decision is made, it must be acted on and then the outcomes evaluated.

3. C: While surveys, observations, and clinical judgment all have a role in developing evidence-based practice, the best approach must include systematic research, generally utilizing online medical databases to find research that supports specific practices. Evidence may be based on basic science, but clinical patient-centered research is preferred. Research should be reviewed carefully to determine if the results have external validity and are generalizable. The CNL utilizes clinical judgment when evaluating research to determine if it is applicable.

4. D: Fentanyl patches are poorly absorbed in cachectic clients because of the lack of adequate muscle and adipose tissue, so the best first action is to switch from fentanyl patches to a long-acting narcotic that can be taken once or twice daily while continuing the OxyContin for breakthrough pain. The client must be carefully monitored during the transition and may initially require increased OxyContin, especially during the first 24 hours. Because the patient has probably not been absorbing all of the dosage of fentanyl, the patient may have increased drowsiness from the oral medication.

5. C: The CNL's primary responsibility is to provide leadership at the point of care. The CNL role was developed to ensure that client care was safe and based on evidence-based research in order to effect positive outcomes. The CNL assists others to make appropriate clinical decisions, to anticipate risks, and to identify preventive measures. The CNL is responsible for evaluating the effectiveness of care, for delegating, and for managing the lateral integration of client care.

6. A: In this case, leadership is evidenced by the CNL taking a course in oncologic pharmacology in preparation for work on an oncology unit. The core role of leadership requires that the CNL serve as a role model to others by advocating for the client, the other members of the healthcare team, and the nursing profession. The CNL must communicate effectively to ensure positive client outcomes. Additionally, the CNL must remain an active professional, pursuing knowledge and remaining current in clinical care.

7. B: The AHRQ Hospital Survey on Patient Safety is a survey designed for hospital staff to gather information about patient safety issues, including medicine errors and reporting of untoward patient events, such as accidents. The survey comprises 9 sections (A-I), which include questions about the unit, the supervisor, communications, frequency of reported events, patient safety grade, the hospital, the number of untoward patient events reported within the previous 12-month period, background information about the surveyed staff, and a comments section. Results can be submitted to the AHRQ database and compared with other facilities.

8. C: With the PFA method, the CNL should first determine the purpose of the search by considering the type of information that needs to be assessed and what the CNL plans to do with the information. The type of search, which is indicated for professional colleagues such as other nurses or team leaders, is a professionally oriented search of medical databases and professional organizations. Government sites and professional organization often provide information specifically intended for professionals.

9. B: This is an example of at-risk behavior. There are 3 classifications using the just culture model:

- Human error: Careless unintentional mistakes and errors, such as failing to double-check a medication dosage.
- At-risk behavior: Risky behavior resulting from failing to follow procedures or failing to recognize a risk exists. These errors result from an incorrect choice.
- Reckless behavior: Consciously committing errors because of disregard for procedures and risks, such as using contaminated equipment or diverting medications.

10. D: The appropriate response to at-risk behavior is coaching:

- Human error: Because these types of errors are common and not intentional, the most appropriate response is to console and support the person who made the error. Processes and procedures should be evaluated to determine if the error resulted from systemic problems.
- At-risk behavior: Because the person ignored safety rules or believed they were not necessary; the person should receive coaching and further training as necessary.
- Reckless behavior: These intentional errors should result in punitive action.

11. A: Distributive: One side wins and the other side loses, also known as zero sum, competitive, or win-lose bargaining. This is the traditional approach to collective bargaining. Integrative: This is a win-win type of bargaining in which both sides attempt to arrive at a mutually acceptable solution. Productivity: Settlement depends on productivity, skills, and knowledge. Composite: Unions negotiate for both salary and standards; for example, the union may want input into work norms and environmental hazards.

12. C: The CNL should confront the team member about violating professional ethics, making clear that the conversation is not appropriate. It's imperative for the CNL to set an example in order to promote an ethical workplace. The organization should have a written code of conduct, which should be communicated to all staff, and all staff should be expected to adhere to the code, including respecting a client's privacy, and should also be expected to confront those who violate the code.

13. B: According to CDC/Healthcare Infection Control Practices Advisory Committee (HICPAC) guidelines to prevent catheter-related infections, insertion sites that are covered with gauze dressings should be palpated every day to evaluate for signs of tenderness, but if there are no signs of infection, the gauze dressing should be left intact and not routinely changed, unless soiled or loosened. If there are indications of infection, the dressing should be removed to allow visual inspection and a new dressing applied. Hand hygiene should be done both before and after palpation of insertion sites.

14. C: The CNL should recommend that the occupational therapist evaluate and instruct the client prior to discharge. After discharge, the patient will probably be faced with food preparation, housework, and child care, so the occupational therapist must carefully evaluate the client's ability to function (swallow, ambulate, dress) and must ensure the client is aware of restrictions, such as no bending over, hot showers, or lifting, as well as the need to sleep with the head elevated.

15. D: Because the client is older than 18 years, he is protected by HIPAA regulations, so the nurse cannot contact the parents, as this would be a violation of privacy. Lecturing clients rarely serves a useful purpose, but doing nothing is not the best solution. Understanding that clients often undergo a period of denial, the CNL recommends that the nurse remain supportive but provide the client with information about the disease and a list of resources.

16. B: The idea that disproportional responses and non-linearity are the norm is part of complexity theory. Patterns are important concepts in complex theory, and a client must be considered in terms of all the relationships and patterns in life that may affect responses and outcomes. Complexity theory suggests that one should not look at a moment in time but consider an event in relation to what comes before and after, and always consider the relationship among many patterns (e.g., emotional, environmental, social, spiritual).

17. C: D5NS is a hypertonic solution and is not appropriate for dehydration, as isotonic solutions are used because they do not cause shifts between extracellular and intracellular compartments. The nurse should immediately contact the physician to question the order. Isotonic fluids, such as normal saline (0.9% sodium chloride), are used to treat volume deficit and dehydration related to vomiting and diarrhea. The client should be carefully monitored during administration of isotonic fluids as hypervolemia may occur quickly.

18. B: While all of these are true, the primary initial concern should be that cross-sensitivity reactions may occur in those with penicillin allergies (about 10%). Therefore, the client should be kept under close observation for at least a half hour after receiving the first dose of cephalexin. Advise the client to call the physician immediately if there are mild symptoms of allergies and 9-1-1 if symptoms are more severe, such as difficulty breathing, or occur suddenly.

19. D: The primary purpose of leader rounding is to improve the relationship between the CNL and team members, so it should never be used for punitive purposes. The CNL should prepare a series of questions to be used with all staff on a regular basis, the frequency depending on the number of staff and time constraints. Questions may include asking what is working well that day, what needs to be improved, whether they have all the tools and equipment they need, if they need any help, and if there is someone on the staff who should be recognized for doing good work.

20. A: Although hospice care is intended for the last 6 months of a person's life, death cannot always be predicted accurately, so the attending physician and medical director of the hospice can certify the client as eligible for hospice care for additional, unlimited 60-day periods. If the client has a change in condition for the better (such as when a client goes into remission from disease), hospice care can be discontinued without penalty and reinstated if the client's condition again becomes terminal.

21. B: The child should receive 1,000 mL plus 100 mL (50 mL for each additional 2 kg of weight) for a total of 1,100 mL of fluid in a 24-hour period. Dividing the total by 24 hours gives the hourly volume of fluid: 1,100/24 = 45.533, rounded to the nearest whole number = 46 mL per hour.

22. D: When using the microdrip system in which 60 drops equal 1 mL, the flow rate will be the same number as the volume per minute. In this case, the flow rate in drops per minute is 46 to administer 46 mL per hour. To calculate, divide the 46 mL by 60 minutes to obtain the fluid volume per minute: 46/60 = 0.7666, rounded to 0.77 mL per minute. Next, multiply the drop factor (60 drops per mL) times the volume per minute (0.77): 60 x 0.77 = 46.2, then round to the nearest whole number, so 46 drops per minute.

23. B: The CMS performance target for door-to-balloon time is 90 minutes or less. This timeframe is indicated for clients presenting with ST-segment elevation myocardial infarction (STEMI) because a delay in percutaneous coronary intervention (PCI) beyond 90 minutes results in severe damage to the heart muscle from inadequate oxygenation, markedly reducing the rate of survival. Emergency department staff must make rapid assessment and contact the catheterization lab, which should be able to perform PCI within 20 to 30 minutes.

24. C: Fixed costs include those costs that are constant and do not fluctuate according to volume or productivity, including administrative salaries, depreciation of buildings and equipment, and utilities. Variable costs can vary widely, depending on client census and other factors. Variable costs include medical supplies, surgical supplies, food costs, and laundry costs. Fixed and variable costs may differ somewhat from one organization to another. For example, nursing costs may be considered a fixed cost if the FTE hours remain the same but may be a variable cost if they vary according to census.

25. D: Staff compliance with best practice guidelines is usually best initially with simple changes in procedures, such as instituting checklists, because the learning curve is rapid and results are generally easily quantified. Because there is no financial outlay for new equipment or need for extensive training, setting up a pilot program is fairly simple. The CNL should provide strong evidence based on research that the new practice is effective and should disseminate the results of a pilot program.

26. A: The CNL should recommend that the patient immediately receive palliative care, which is intended to help patients relieve symptoms of disease and to provide emotional, spiritual, and physical support. While palliative care is one aspect of hospice care, it is appropriate throughout the course of an illness. Even though the patient is receiving aggressive therapy, issues such as pain control, diet, nausea, and elimination are common, and dealing with these issues can improve the client's quality of life.

27. C: Perceived susceptibility is the degree to which a person believes he or she is susceptible to a condition. If a person's perceived susceptibility is low regarding the chances of developing diabetes or heart disease, the person is less likely to make necessary changes. Perceived severity is the person's perception of the seriousness of the condition and associated consequences. Perceived benefit is the person's belief in the effectiveness of action, and perceived barriers are the perception of costs (emotional, spiritual, financial) related to an action.

28. C: According to Pender's Health Promotion Model, interpersonal influences can have a profound effect on clients' compliance with health promotion and preventive measures. Even when clients recognize their susceptibility and understand the severity of risk and benefits of compliance, they may be unwilling to risk relationships and may feel that the benefits, emotional or otherwise, derived from their social groups outweighs the benefits of change. The CNL must always consider personal factors, such as interpersonal influences, when working with clients and others to facilitate change.

29. D: Under de Bono's Six Thinking Hats technique, the Blue Hat facilitates the discussion and provides structure so that the other six "thinking" hats are utilized properly. The White Hat provides objective facts and figures to help the group understand what information they have. The Red Hat deals with positive and negative emotions. The Yellow Hat looks for positive aspects while the Black Hat serves as the devil's advocate, challenging assumptions. The Green Hat provides creative and innovative solutions.

30. A: An example of a normative re-educative strategy to facilitate and manage change is to encourage the team to identify problems and solutions because this causes them to become active participants in the process of change. While this method of facilitating change may take longer than the empirical-rational model, which relies on facts and figures to bring about rational decisions, or the power-coercive strategy, which enforces change with power, it is often the most successful.

31. D: Resistance to change is very common, so ignoring the resistant team members, calling them out, or punishing them can be counterproductive. The best solution is to ask the resistant team members to take active roles in facilitating change, empowering them and developing trust. People often resist change because they are unsure how the change will affect them personally, especially if they believe that they will lose some degree of control over their actions or decision-making.

32. A: Low-context cultures (such as the United States, Canada, Northern Europe, Russia, and England) rely on written or spoken word to carry meaning, while high-context cultures (such as Asian countries, Saudi Arabia, Pacific Islands, and Mexico) rely on context and situation to carry meaning rather than words. People from high-context cultures may have difficulty answering directly and may feel uncomfortable and challenged by direct questions, while those from low-context cultures may feel the others are frustrating and evasive.

33. D: Computerized physician order entry (CPOE) systems provide the safest method for physicians to order medications because there is no problem with legibility. The programs include safeguards and can provide alerts if an order is incomplete or dosage incorrect. Some systems, for example, also provide alerts if interactions may occur between two medications. Most systems have links that provide drug information, including information about adverse effects. The Institute of Medicine (IOM) recommends eliminating handwritten orders to prevent medication errors.

34. A: While generational differences may hold true for a group, they do not necessarily apply to an individual in that group. However, the CNL is probably more comfortable with new technology because Millennials (born 1981-1999) grew up with computers, video games, and other electronic equipment and feel comfortable multi-tasking and using electronic equipment to access information and carry out tasks. Members of the Silent Generation (born 1925-1945) usually have respect for authority while Baby Boomers (born 1946-1964) tend to question authority. Generation Xers (born 1965-1980) are likely to be skeptical of traditional practices.

35. C: Professional advocacy includes actions that increase the visibility, legitimacy, and viability of the profession, such as the CNL clarifying the role of CNL within an organization or lobbying for improvements in healthcare within the community. Other examples of professional advocacy include involvement in local, state, and national organizations. The CNL advocates for the profession by explaining the CNL role to others, by supporting political issues relevant to nursing, and by serving as a role model for other staff members.

36. D: Indirect patient care functions, such as leadership, staff management, operations, and research, are critical to ensure that direct patient care functions, such as patient education, coordination of care, and communication, are effective. The CNL—as leader of a team—is responsible for both indirect and direct patient care functions, but the CNL must delegate direct patient care functions to ensure that all clients receive the necessary care. The CNL should also delegate indirect patient care functions in order to develop leadership abilities in staff members.

37. A: In the event of a disaster, increasing surge capacity allows for admission of large number of injured clients. The initial strategy is to identify clients safely eligible for early discharge. This may also include cancelling scheduled procedures, such as elective surgeries. Extra beds can be placed in outpatient areas and in hallways, as this is more time-effective than attempting to transfer existing patients to different rooms and cleaning and preparing the rooms. In some cases, nondisaster-related clients may be diverted to other hospitals, but in most cases, other facilities will also be impacted by the disaster.

38. C: Suprasystems are those systems outside of the immediate environment of the facility, such as accrediting agencies and public health systems, but suprasystems may have a profound effect on the facility.

Most systems are comprised of a number of subsystems. For a hospital, subsystems might include laboratory services, security, and housekeeping. Because systems within a hospital exchange information and staff, they are considered open systems. Closed systems, which function completely independently, are rare.

39. D: According to the STAR model, a change in one area usually necessitates a change in another area because of the interrelatedness of systems. The STAR model is based on a diagram with the points of the STAR representing strategy, structure, human resources, incentives, and information/decision making. Values that are core to this model include the idea that a systemic problem is rarely related to laziness or incompetence, there are multiple optimal systems, many points are equally important, and cultures or values may be ingrained, impeding progress, and cannot be changed directly.

40. B: According to the Systems Theory (Bertalanffy), an expected output would be improved client care and outcomes. The 5 elements of the theory are (1) input, the energy or materials (nurses and clients) that go into a system; (2) throughput, the actions taken to transform input (managing and supervising); (3) output, the result of the throughput on input (improved client outcomes); (4) evaluation, determining if the throughput was effective; and (5) feedback. This theory views the system holistically, recognizing that all parts of the system are interrelated.

41. B: According to the CNL Standards of Conduct, altruism is concern for and advocating for the welfare of clients and staff and demonstrating understanding of others' beliefs and values. Accountability is using rights and power to act competently. Integrity is carrying out practice in an ethical manner and according to standards of practice. Social justice is ensuring patients are treated in accordance with the laws regarding access to care in a fair manner without discrimination. Human dignity is showing respect for the individual and populations, respecting privacy and confidentiality, and providing culturally competent care.

42. D: The best way to communicate changes in processes to team members is to utilize multiple and repeated means of communication; telling staff members one time or in one manner is rarely sufficient because some staff may not be paying close attention and other staff may be resistive. The CNL may post the information, make an announcement, discuss the matter with individual staff persons, and then remind staff frequently during team meetings, evaluating progress toward the change.

43. C: A communication board must be updated on a regular basis if it is to remain relevant; otherwise, staff members won't bother to read it. The CNL should plan to update the communication board on a weekly schedule, preferably on the same day so that staff members can predict when to look for new information. Communication boards often have information organized into categories, such as *service, quality, staff, economics, growth, community,* and *news.* The communication board should be placed in an area with easy access for staff.

44. A: The most important factor for the CNL to communicate to staff when proposing changes in processes and procedures is the reason because staff members are more likely to be cooperative if they understand why they are asked to make changes. The CNL should be prepared to present evidence-based rationale for changes and to discuss anticipated outcomes so that the staff fully understands that the changes are not arbitrary and that they should result in positive results.

45. B: A rounding log—a signed record of staff client visits kept at the point of care—is primarily intended to improve client outcomes by ensuring that the staff interacts with the client on a regular basis, usually at least every hour. This allows staff to more carefully observe changes in a client's condition and reassures the client that staff is concerned about his/her welfare. The rounding log serves as a reminder to staff that all clients are in need of care and attention.

46. A: Because inappropriate and unprofessional behavior is a serious matter that may result in client legal action and/or punitive action toward the staff person, the CNL should consult with human resources to make sure that proper protocol is followed. All interactions should be carefully documented, including the complaints and any interventions. Human resources can advise the CNL about issues related to privacy and confidentiality and, in many cases, may assume responsibility for dealing with the problem.

47. D: Intuitive thinking: A "gut" or intuitive feeling that something is wrong (or right) despite having no objective basis for the feeling. Experienced nurses often develop intuitive thinking based on subtle clues. Critical thinking: Evaluating the processes of thought and decision-making to ensure positive outcomes. This may involve carrying out specific steps in a decision-making process. Reflective thinking: Observing and assessing one's own thought processes. Problem solving: Actively seeking a solution to a specific problem.

48. B: The DESK model follows this model:

- Describe the problem behavior so the staff person understands exactly what behavior has been observed and needs correction.
- Explain how the problem behavior affects client outcomes or unit performance.
- Show the staff person exactly what steps the person needs to take to improve performance. This may include counseling, coaching, and re-educating.
- Know the consequences: The staff person should be aware of what will happen if he or she fails to make necessary changes

49. C: Research indicates that a 3:1 ratio of recognition to criticism is essential to maintaining a positive culture. While the CNL does not need to count and keep a record to ensure this ratio, it's good to remember that positive recognition is just as important as criticism because leaders often neglect to give positive feedback overtly, assuming that team members realize they are doing well if they receive no criticism, but an absence of criticism does not mean that team members feel valued.

50. A: Behavioral interviewing requires open-ended questions, such as "Tell me about a time when..." This type of question results in a narrative answer. Utilizing the EAR model to record the interviewees' answers, the CNL will record the event that took place, the action that the interviewees carried out to resolve the issue presented by the event, and the results of the action. This is an organized method of taking notes and is especially helpful when interviewing multiple candidates.

51. D: If the CNL is ceding the authority to hire to a peer interview team, then the CNL should only pick candidates that the CNL would be willing to hire because peer dynamics are often different than those between a leader and staff, and the peer group may have different priorities. While picking only those with the best qualifications may sound like a good plan, qualifications alone do not determine whether a person will be a good team member or not.

52. B: The only legal question is, "Would you have a problem working a 12-hour shift?" The CNL may not legally ask any question about age, including the year of graduation from nursing school, and may not inquire about disabilities, although it is legal to ask what accommodations might be needed after someone is hired. Any personal questions, such as about living situations, family, sexual orientation, or religion, are illegal. All questions should stay focused on job performance and job requirements.

53. B: The CNL should ask a high-performing member of the team to serve as a mentor. This serves the double purpose of orienting the newly hired team member and developing leadership skills in the mentor. The CNL should communicate with both the newly hired team member and the mentor frequently to note progress and offer support and guidance. Mentoring relationship may vary in length of time, depending on the complexity of the work environment, but 6 months to a year is common.

54. D: The nursing process is very similar to the process of education and can be used to describe the different elements of instruction. The nursing process focuses on plans and action related to the patient diagnosis, while the education process focuses on plans and actions related to learner needs:

- Assess: Assess learning needs and styles and readiness to learn.
- Plan: Develop teaching plans with associated outcomes.
- Implement: Carry out instruction using different tools and teaching strategies.
- Evaluate: Evaluate outcomes, including changes in behavior based on proposed outcomes.

55. A: A flow chart is used to present a process schematically and is often used to analyze processes as part of quality improvement. A flow chart may be used to help visualize a proposed process as well as current processes. Typically, standardized symbols are used in the chart:

- Parallelogram: Input and output (start/end).
- Arrow: Direction of flow.
- Diamond shape: Conditional decision (Yes/No or True/False).
- Circles: Connectors with multiple arrows from divergent paths coming into the circle but only one going out.

56. B: The fact that 6 out of 30 clients needed to use the call bell to ask for pain medications indicates that care related to pain management is inadequate as staff should be proactive in assessing clients for pain, evaluating their pain levels, and offering pain medication as ordered. Control of pain allows clients to move more actively and recover more quickly. Staff may need further training on the 3 Ps (pain, potty, and position), which should be addressed routinely.

57. C: The most effective initial intervention is likely to be pre-visit telephone calls a day or two prior to surgery to remind clients of the time and any preparation needed and also to reassure them and ask if they have any questions or concerns. Clients should be advised to come at least a half hour prior to their scheduled time so that paperwork can be completed and clients admitted to the unit. The clients should be encouraged to ask questions and to write down any questions they might have for the physician and to bring the questions with them.

58. A: If team members are properly conducting hourly nursing rounds and asking patients about their pain and bathroom needs, helping them change position, and asking if they need assistance in any other way, there should be a marked reduction in the number of call bells as these are the primary reasons that people use the call bell. If the number of calls is stored in the system, that information can be easily retrieved. Otherwise, a count should be kept for a specified period of time (a week to a month) before and after instituting hourly rounds.

59. D: The greatest risk to an organization's computer network security is from malicious insiders, such as a recently fired employee or a disgruntled employee who wants to cause problems for the organization. Most organizations now utilize software that tracks employee activity and separates privileges so that one employee cannot independently carry out an action that could result in a critical breach. When an employee is fired or leaves employment, that person's access code must be immediately deactivated.

60. C: Information gathered about events, such as patient falls without injury and patient falls with injury, is best differentiated by unit if used to facilitate quality improvement. While differentiating by the organization allows comparisons with similar organizations, it doesn't help to pinpoint weak areas within the organization. In some cases, a high-performing unit with no falls will dilute the results and mask a unit with a large number of falls, so differentiating by unit allows the organization to analyze the problems that may be resulting in falls.

61. B: The most efficient method of reminding staff members to carry out client education, such as the need for immunizations, is to imbed the prompts in the clinical information system/electronic health record. A prompt may ask if the teaching has been completed and should, for example, link to specific detailed information about immunizations, including type and frequency for the client's age and condition. The prompts should appear with each access of the record until the staff members responds that the teaching has been completed.

62. B: The data mart is a smaller component of the larger data warehouse. A data warehouse is generally a huge database that contains all of the data of an organization and is available for data mining. A data mart contains all of the information of a smaller area, such as one unit or one healthcare system. For example, if there are a number of associated hospitals represented in the database, each may have a separate data mart housing its individual data.

63. C: Background includes current vital signs and descriptions of pain. SBAR is a technique commonly used for hand-off procedures to make sure that all important information is conveyed. Elements include:

- Situation: Name, age, MD, diagnosis.
- Background: Brief medical history, co-morbidities, review of lab tests, current therapy, IVs, VS, pain, special needs, educational needs, discharge plans.
- Assessment: Review of systems, lines, tubes, and drains, completed tasks, needed tasks, future procedures.
- Recommendations: Review plan of care, medications, precautions (restraints, falls), treatments, wound care.

64. A: The initial step in IPC is to identify what is important to the client: "What three things can we do to make sure you receive excellent care?" The CNL may ask specific questions if the client has no response. The client's list should be written on a whiteboard or posted in the client's room so that everyone who goes into the room reviews them. At each round and shift change, the list should be addressed to find out if the client's needs are being met. They should be reviewed again on discharge and in the discharge survey.

65. D: Acknowledgment refers to acknowledging the person, using the person's name. Adults should generally be addressed by their surname, such as "Mrs. Smith," rather than the less formal first name unless the client has specifically asked to be addressed by the first name. Introduce includes introducing oneself to the client and explaining one's position and the treatment. Duration explains how long the treatment will take. Explanation includes the reason the treatment is being carried out. Thanks is explicitly stated to the client.

66. B: In a service recovery model, the first step is acknowledging the problem and apologizing for the inconvenience to the client: "I know you have been kept waiting for an hour, and I'm so sorry for the delay." The next step is to attempt to correct the situation. The following step is to make amends in some way, which may include providing some type of compensation (gift card, cup of coffee). The last step is to take action to prevent a repetition of the problem in the future.

67. D: The CNL should understand the need for the client to vent frustration but must also set acceptable parameters for behavior: "I would like to help you, but first I need to understand what the problem is." Once the client provides this information, the nurse should avoid placing blame or making excuses, but should apologize. The next step is to find out from the client what would repair the damage: "What can I do to make you feel better?" and try to provide more than what the client expects.

68. A: While improved client care is always important, senior management is often most concerned with financial obligations, so the best approach for the CNL is generally to focus on cost-effectiveness, showing how an extra staff person may result in reduced overall costs because of fewer infections and falls and better client satisfaction, which brings loyalty to the institution. While the goal of the CNL may be client-focused, the CNL frames the request in terms of cost savings.

69. C: "Cost shifting" is essentially shifting costs for lost income to others, such as when the hospital increases ED costs to private pay and insured clients to offset loss from those with no insurance or means to pay. This is an increasingly common problem as hospitals try to find creative ways to offset financial losses, sometimes resulting in costs that seem exorbitant but are, in fact, paid by only a small number of clients.

70. B: While leaving extra linen in clients' rooms is a common practice to save team members the time it takes to go procure linen, it is not a cost-effective practice. Much of the linen is likely to be unused when clients are discharged, and this extra linen must then be sent to the laundry, adding to the costs for water, soap, and disinfectant, as well as staff time needed to process the extra linen and restock linen supply cabinets.

71. C: Eleven FTEs are employed each week. One FTE is equivalent to 40 hours (2,080 annually) so full-time (40-hour) staff each equals one FTE while the 4 part-time (20-hour) RNs are each 0.5 FTE. When calculating FTEs, it's important to remember that hours, not staff members, must be counted. FTEs are usually calculated on an annual basis and must include paid vacation and sick time because those hours are budgeted for, but must also account for any unpaid leave as those hours are not counted.

72. D: Worked hours per patient day (WHPPD) are budgeted according to projections of the number of hours of direct client care a nurse will provide in 24 hours. Budgeted hours may vary (usually from 7 to 16), depending on the unit. The goal is productivity of 95% to 105%. Since 8 hours were budgeted but 10 hours of direct client care were required, 8/10 = 80% productivity. Very high productivity (fewer hours needed than those budgeted) may increase risks to clients while low productivity (more hours needed than those budgeted) results in increased costs to the organization.

73. A: Rankings may be calculated with various measures, including raw scores and mean/average scores, but for comparison purposes, when looking at benchmarks, percentile ranking is often utilized. A score of 69% indicates that this unit scored better than 69% of those the unit was benchmarking against. Score may be classified as being in the top decile (10%) or quartile (25%) as well. The goal is generally to score at least at the 50% ranking and to steadily increase percentile rankings.

74. D: *Hospital Compare* reports only the top box score—it only reports the results for the highest possible rating. In this case, the reported score is 72%. Because the range of scores is not reported, this can skew scores. For example, if one hospital scored 50% for always and 48% for usually, 2% for sometimes, and 0% for never, and another scored 65% for always, 10% for usually, 10% for sometimes, and 5% for never, the first hospital actually is more successful but the second hospital would score considerably higher. Therefore, the goal is 100% compliance.

75. C: The initial step for the CNL should be to filter the surveys by shift to try to pinpoint whether there is a difference in scores from one shift to another, as is often the case. This can help the CNL target strategies to improve outcomes. Staff may provide a variety of different reasons why they believe test scores are low, but they often are not really sure or blame various factors, such as inadequate staff.

76. C: With the nominal group technique, the group leader presents an issue or poses a question and then the group begins by silently considering the issue and writing out ideas without discussion. The next step is for each member to present his or her ideas, including any advantages and disadvantages. The following step is for the group to discuss, evaluate, and discuss the ideas that were presented. Finally, the last step is to privately vote to determine which idea has the majority support.

77. A: The primary advantage of the Delphi decision-making technique is that group members don't have to actually meet face to face. This makes the technique ideal for large groups. The CNL or group leader creates a questionnaire and then distributes it to all group members, who respond and return the questionnaire. The results are tabulated and summarized and returned to participants. This process may be repeated multiple times until the group reaches consensus.

78. D: *D* stands for *date of last update*. The PLEASED technique comprises:

P—Purpose: The author's purpose in developing the site as well as the researcher's purpose in accessing the site.
L—Links: Live links as opposed to dead links, types of links, and quality of links.
E—Editorial: Accuracy and bias, grammar, and structure.
A—Author: Identification and credentials.
S—Site navigation: Ease of navigation and use, structure.
E—Ethical disclosures: Contact information and other disclosures, such as employment.
D—Date of last update: Current or out-of-date.

79. D: The CNL should suggest that the nurse administer use the Confusion Assessment Method because these signs and symptoms are indicative of delirium. The tool covers 9 factors associated with delirium: rapid onset, attention, disorganized thinking, altered consciousness, disorientation, impaired memory, perceptual disturbances, psychomotor abnormalities, and disturbance in sleep-wake cycle. MMSE and Mini-Cog are used to evaluate cognitive impairment and dementia. The Palliative Performance Scale is used to assess functional abilities in those receiving palliative care.

80. C: Medications used to reduce the symptoms of delirium include trazodone, lorazepam, and haloperidol. A sitter should also be provided to ensure the client's safety as he may try to climb out of bed in his confused state. If the client is receiving hypnotics or psychotropics, dosages should be reduced. Delirium occurs in 10% to 40% of hospitalized older adults and 80% of terminally ill clients. Some medications (anticholinergics) and conditions (hypoxia, infection, hearing loss, vision loss, uncontrolled pain, and fluid/electrolyte imbalance) may trigger delirium.

81. C: The CNL should anticipate most members would be classified as *proficient*. Benner's model:

- Novice: Little or no experience, rule-oriented, and task-focused. Needs mentoring.
- Advanced beginner: 1-2 years of experience, better able to rely on principles related to experience but benefits from mentoring.
- Competent: 2-3 years of experience, more adept at critical thinking and planning and increasingly efficient.
- Proficient: 3-5 years of experience, able to look at situations holistically rather than at tasks and has improved decision-making based on experience.
- Expert: 5-10 years of experience, relieves on intuitive thinking as well as critical thinking and can adapt well to new situations and is adept at decision-making.

82. B: The best answer explains where the value in leadership experience lies: "Leadership skills will help you be more effective when working with clients, other nurses, and unlicensed assistive personnel." Leadership is a process that results in the person having influence over others. Even a novice nurse interacts with many people—including clients and other team members—so nurses at all levels of experience need leadership skills, even if their immediate goal is not that of management.

83. A: According to the Contingency Theory (a behavioral approach), successful leadership is contingent on many factors, including individuals, situations, resources, and organizational culture. What works well in one situation may not apply equally to another, so a leader needs to be flexible and should thoroughly assess all factors before deciding on a course of action or management style. Significant changes are best managed in small incremental steps when possible, so the CNL may need to gradually work toward a democratic style of leadership in the new environment.

84. B: With horizontal leadership, the CNL would share information directly with other teams rather than going through the time-consuming process involved in a more hierarchical structure in which information is sent upward, approved, and then sent back down through the chain of command. Horizontal leadership usually involves fewer middle managers, and exchange of information among peer groups is encouraged, allowing staff members to more readily communicate and share data and information at the points of care.

85. B: Native Americans have the lowest life expectancy of any ethnic group in the United States, with a life expectancy that is only two-thirds that of other groups. Native Americans also have the highest rate of poverty (30%). They include 5.2 million people who identify as Native American/Alaskan Native or mixed race. Native Americans/Alaska Natives are increasing in number with an increase of almost 27% from 2000 to 2010, while the overall population grew only about 10%. Approximately 22% of Native American/Alaska Natives live in federal or state reservations while the remaining live among the general population. Less than 0.5% of nurses are Native American/Alaska Native.

86. A: Juran's quality improvement process begins with the CNL listing and prioritizing problems as well as defining the problem and creating an improvement process team, which in some cases may be an existing team. The next step is to diagnose the problem by analyzing them and trying to identify cause through root cause analysis and to test theories. The following step is to remediate the problems by considering various methods to resolve problems and designing specific solutions and controls. Finally, the team holds the gains achieved by these interventions through evaluation and monitoring.

87. B: The "Five Whys" method begins with the problem: "Why did the client climb over the bedrails?" The answer then generates the next question. For example, if the answer is that the client could not reach the call bell, the next question would be, "Why couldn't the client reach the call bell?" This process, designed by Ohno for Toyota in Japan, seeks to find the root cause of a problem by asking a series of at least 5 questions. Once consensus is reached, team members propose solutions to improve performance.

88. C: The data collection that is most indicated to measure outcomes to determine if teaching is effective is readmission data. Clients with respiratory disorders, such as chronic asthma and COPD, have frequent hospitalizations if they are not able to manage their disease symptoms, so interventions that teach clients better self-care should impact readmission rates. A timeframe should be determined—usually at least a period of a few months—based on the frequency of readmissions prior to the intervention.

89. B: A method of quantitative data collection is conducting interviews asking each participant the exact same questions with no variation, such as yes/no or multiple choice questions, because the results can be easily tabulated. Questionnaires may be utilized instead of interviews and may include checklists and rating scales. Open-ended questions may yield different answers for each participant, so the results may be summarized but not accurately quantified. Observations are by nature qualitative data because they rely on subjective assessment.

90. D: Provider-focused outcomes are those related to the people delivering care, such as nurses. Measures can include nurse turnover rates and job satisfaction surveys. Client/Patient focused outcomes may relate to diseases and conditions, pain management, patient satisfaction, symptom control, preventive measures, and readmission rates. Organization-focused outcomes relate to the organization as a whole and may include mortality rates and cost indicators. Patient-focused and provider-focused outcomes may be aggregated and considered as part of organization-focused outcomes.

91. A: Protective factors include knowledge about the risks of substance abuse and negative attitudes toward use, as well as social competence, self-confidence, and good relationships with at least some adults. Predictive factors include poor reading and academic skills, early sexual activity, uncertainty about future plans, inherited tendency, history of psychological and psychiatric disorders, history of violence, lack of social skills, early behavioral problems, and association with substance abusers.

92. D: Almost (2005) classified antecedents of conflict as related to three things:

- Interpersonal factors: These include lack of trust, lack of respect, injustice, unfairness, and poor communication.
- Individual characteristics: Value differences, different opinions, and gender and ethnic differences.
- Organizational factors: Restructuring, change, and interdependence.

Other researchers consider professional differences a separate cause for conflict. These may occur when different professionals have opposing points of view about treatment plans or have different levels of education.

93. C: The CNL is faced with a situation in which two team members have different communication strategies, resulting in conflict. The best solution is one that retains both team members: conflict resolution. The CNL must remain neutral and listen to both sides present their sides of the conflict and then help them arrive at a compromise that will allow cooperation. The CNL should avoid forcing resolution but can point out their differences in communication and ask the two to explain to each other how they felt during the confrontation.

94. A: Cost-benefit analysis is used to compare the average cost of an event and the cost of intervention to demonstrate savings. For example, if each stage IV pressure sore costs the hospital an additional $125,000 and the hospital averages 6 stage IV pressure sores each year, the annual cost is $750,000. If an additional staff member specializing in wound care costs $120,000 (including benefits) and better wound treatment costs an additional $28,000 per year, the cost of intervention is $148,000. The cost-benefit is then $750,000 minus $148,000 = $602,000 in savings.

95. B: Hospital B is likely to receive the most reimbursement for services because its payor mix has fewer Medicare and Medicaid patients. Medicaid, for example, usually pays about half of the reimbursement rate of private insurers. Medicare also generally pays considerably less. Hospital B has 36% of patients receiving coverage from insurance compared with only 8% at hospital A. Additionally, hospital B has fewer uninsured patients, and these costs must often be absorbed by the hospitals.

96. C: The CDC recommends that indwelling urinary catheters be used only when absolutely necessary and not be used to treat incontinence unless the patient has an open perineal or sacral wound that may worsen with contact with urine. Catheters inserted for long surgical procedures should be removed in the recovery area. Catheters are still recommended for acute urinary retention or conditions that may result in bladder distention, such as bladder outlet obstruction. Catheters may also be necessary for critically ill clients when fluid balance must be carefully monitored.

97. B: Fixed or forecast budgets are based on estimated revenue and costs and budget items are fixed so that additions cannot be made to the budget during the budget period. Zero-based budgets require that each cost center be re-evaluated each budget period and the budget built again from zero. Rolling/Continuous budgets have periodic updates to the budget depending on costs and revenue during the budget period. Flexible budgets account for both fixed costs and variable costs with estimates based on anticipated changes in costs and revenue.

98. D: The CNL's *span of control* refers to the number of staff persons who report to the CNL. If the span of control is narrow, then the CNL is responsible for supervising a small number of staff persons, but this can increase costs. However, if the span of control is too broad, the CNL may not be able to adequately fulfill duties and adequately supervise and lead. The span of control should be balanced so that the CNL can effectively lead and remain cost-effective.

99. B: The usual purpose of a clinical practice partnership council is to establish nursing practice standards. Partnership councils may exist at different levels within an organization, so there may be central partnership councils as well as unit councils. Each organization may have many different councils with different areas of responsibility. Partnership councils are more inclusive than earlier forms of shared governance. Partnership councils may include staff persons from all levels/areas within an organization rather than solely nursing personnel, a recognition that all staff persons contribute to the organization's mission.

100. A: SWOT analysis is most commonly used to develop a strategic plan for an organization. SWOT analysis considers the Strengths and Weaknesses of the internal environment and the Opportunities and Threats of the external environment:

Internal environment		External environment	
Strengths	**Weaknesses**	**Opportunities**	**Threats**
Financial stability	Increasing costs	Increased population	Low reimbursement
Programs, services	Outdated equipment	New programs	Regulations
Staff persons	Ineffective programs	New markets	Competition
Client/staff satisfaction	Marketing	Stakeholders	Political changes

101. D: Divergent thinking allows for a number of diverse ideas, often generated through the brainstorming process in which various possible solutions are proposed and discussed. Ideas should be expressed spontaneously without judgment. This may be followed by the more rule-oriented convergent thinking, during which ideas are organized and the best possible solution identified. Divergent thinking focuses on various possibilities while convergent thinking focuses on probabilities, or the one best solution to a problem.

102. D: Being found grossly negligent in caring for a client is grounds for sanctions against the CNL by the Commission on Nurse Certification. Other grounds include:

- Violating the Standards of Conduct.
- Being convicted of a felony or crime of moral turpitude related to nursing practice.
- Falsely supplying information on original application.
- Falsifying any information requested by the Board.
- Misrepresenting nursing status.
- Cheating on certification examinations.
- Sanctions may include being reprimanded or suspended or having license revoked.

103. B: Patient safety is the primary concern of risk management in healthcare today because the best cost-saving measure is to prevent errors that lead to negative client outcomes. Risk management developed as a profession in the 1970s in response to increased claims for malpractice that resulted in huge, financially devastating settlements. Since then, the role of risk management has shifted from reactive to proactive, and risk managers have become advocates for patient safety and preventive measures.

104. C: The next action should be to conduct root-cause analysis to try to determine the reason for the increased rate of central line–associated infections. Root-cause analysis is carried out after events to determine causes. The process may involve interviews, observations, and reviews of medical records. Root-cause analysis attempts to identify problems in processes and systems that result in error rather than individuals. Once a problem has been identified, process improvement plans should be initiated based on literature review and best practices.

105. B: The CNL should help the team leader develop an action plan to improve leadership skills and should begin by focusing on the leader's strengths, such as her organization skills and her leadership potential. The CNL may ask the team leader to take a leadership assessment so the team leader can better understand her own approach to leadership. The action plan should include specific steps, such as the team leader making a point of asking for input from each team member at each shift.

106. A: Magnet status requires a participative/collaborative management style that allows for feedback from staff members at all levels in an organization. The organizational structure must be flat and decentralized with staff members at the unit level able to make decisions that apply to their work area. The chief nursing officer must be a member of the executive team and report to the chief executive officer of the organization. The organization must pay competitive salaries and offer flexible staffing models. All nurses must participate in quality improvement processes, and interdisciplinary relationships must be positive.

107. D: In states or organizations that mandate a specific nurse to patient ratio, generally the only circumstances under which the ratio can be bypassed is a health emergency, such as a disaster or epidemic. Federal law requires "adequate numbers" of licensed nursing personnel but does not specify an exact ratio, but nursing organizations have supported minimum levels. As of 2014, 13 states have enacted laws related to staffing. Some states require disclosure of nurse to patient ratio, some require organizations to have staffing committees to establish ratios, and California specifies exact nurse to patient ratios ranging from 1:1 to 1:6.

108. C: When calculating nurse to patient ratios, generally only licensed nurses providing direct patient care are considered. Unlicensed assistive personnel are excluded as are nurse managers not providing direct patient care. Licensed nurses include both RNs and LPNs/LVNs but some states or organizations may restrict the number of LPNs/LVNs that may be counted or may not allow LPNs/LVNs to work in some specialty areas. These are important staffing considerations when determining an effective ratio and maintaining cost-effectiveness.

109. C: Because many organizations scan resumes, the CNL should avoid a two-column format, as the columns may become jumbled during the scanning process. The CNL should be sure to include as many key words as possible from the job description in the resume because those that have the most matches are usually selected. The CNL should use a plain type font and may highlight using bolding or capital letters but should avoid dashes, underlining, and parentheses.

110. A: The primary measure of quality practice for a CNL is improved clinical and cost outcomes. Each organization should set its own measures, which may include decreased hospital-associated infections, decreased hospital-acquired pressure sores, decreased falls, increased staff and/or client satisfaction, and decreased patient stays with outcomes compared with internal and external benchmarks. A monetary value may be placed on many of these measures, so the cost-effectiveness of the CNL position may be determined as well as the improvement in clinical outcomes.

111. B: The CNL should base clinical practice guidelines on evidence. Evidence-based practice is absolutely central to the work of the CNL, who should keep up with the latest research by reading journals and accessing information in medical databases. The CNL should present evidence when proposing changes and when rounding with staff and serve as a role model for team members. The

CNL should review practices and processes in terms of current research, always seeking more effective ways to provide care.

112. D: New graduates often have had little or no experience caring for dying clients or working with the families and may feel insecure and unsure of how to react or how to be supportive. In this instance, the best approach is for the CNL to practice role-playing with the nurse. The nurse should understand the importance of acknowledging the family and can practice simple phrases to offer comfort. The nurse may find it easier to offer a service, such as a warm blanket, pillow, or coffee, and this is a good way to show support.

113. C: The most important factor in ensuring clients participate fully in care is health literacy. It's not enough to teach clients procedures; they must also understand underlying health issues, risk factors, and preventive measures. The nurse must assess a client's understanding and tailor education to the client's needs. The client should know where to go to find information, which organizations might address the client's disease or injury, and what resources are available in the community.

114. A: In the future, Medicare payments as well as insurance payments will be increasingly performance-based so that compensation is tied to performance measures that must be achieved. A number of pilot programs are currently using this system, also known as pay-for-performance (P4P) and value-based purchasing. Healthcare providers are paid incentives for reaching goals. Some states already have P4P plans in effect, and it is an element of the Affordable Care Act. Current plans are that 9% of Medicare payments will be performance based by 2017.

115. B: When a client is admitted to an acute care hospital under the Medicare Inpatient Prospective Payment System (IPPS), clients must be given a present on admission (POA) Medicare Severity Diagnosis Related Group (MS-DRG) diagnosis, which includes all primary and secondary diagnoses. If conditions are not noted on admission but noted on discharge, Medicare will assume the condition was acquired during hospitalization and will not pay. Medicare also will not pay if the condition is present on discharge and documentation is not adequate to determine if it was present on admission.

116. C: Because errors are most often related to a problem with process rather than individuals, the CNL should begin by reviewing admission procedures and admission forms. In most cases, nurses follow the format laid out by the admission forms, so the CNL should determine exactly how the form questions skin integrity and whether the form needs clarification or the addition of a checklist. The CNL should also assess data to determine if other POA diagnoses may have been missed. The CNL should also evaluate the timeframe associated with the admission procedure.

117. B: The Joint Commission's National Patient Safety Goals for Ambulatory Care (2014) includes four categories: identifying patients correctly, using medicines safely, preventing infection, and preventing mistakes in surgery. The 3 steps in the latter category are 1) ensure surgery is on the correct client and correct body part, (2) mark the correct place on the client's body, and (3) pause before surgery to ensure mistakes aren't being made. While the guidelines don't specify the use of a checklist, many organizations use checklists to ensure that no steps have been overlooked.

118. A: The CNL should survey best practices and OSHA regulations and promote establishment of a comprehensive safe client handling program that includes not only extensive staff training in body mechanics and lifting techniques but also the proper use of assistive equipment. The CNL should advocate for more and better equipment to facilitate lifting and transferring clients. According to OSHA, the costs associated with back injuries to healthcare workers is estimated to be about $20 billion each year, and up to a fifth of nurses leave direct care positions because of risks associated with client care.

119. D: The two elements that are essential for a nurse and client to establish a therapeutic alliance are mutuality and reciprocity. Mutuality is a sharing between the nurse and client, such as when they are both working toward a mutual goal. The nurse and client must directly or indirectly mutually agree on the degree of interpersonal involvement and must practice reciprocity so that an action on one's part brings about a response on the other.

120. A: Holistic assessment: Focus is on gaining a broad perspective on a client's problems and concerns and factors, such as social history, that may impact recovery. Problem-focused assessment: The focus is on assessing the status of an already identified problem. Emergency assessment: The focus is on rapidly assessing a client in situations that are life-threatening, such as suicide attempt or accident, MI, or stroke. Ongoing assessment: Focus is on conducting an assessment at a time period after the initial assessment to determine if changes have occurred.

121. C: The epidemiological triad comprises the agent, host, and environment. The CNL must often use epidemiological approaches to problem solving and reducing risk factors. He or she should have a clear understanding of epidemiological principles before beginning to collect data:

- Agent: Organism (virus, bacterium, fungus).
- Host: Receiver of the agent, resulting in infection.
- Environment: Place or conditions under which an agent is able to infect a host.

The information gleaned from epidemiological research can be used not just to identify causes and errors but also to facilitate change.

122. A: Journals that require that articles be juried have rigorous standards for research, so when researching best practices, they provide the most valid resources. However, useful information may be gained from other sources, such as online sites (WebMD.com, Mayoclinic.org, Medicinenet.com), but the findings should be verified by other sources. Physicians, such as Dr. Oz, who serve as TV personalities and "experts," may provide useful information but it may be outside of their area of expertise and may be anecdotal rather than supported by research.

123. B: Screening Tool of Older Persons' potentially inappropriate Prescriptions (STOPP) provides lists of medications that are potentially inappropriate for those 65 years and older because of the danger of adverse reactions. STOPP has 65 criteria, organized by body system, describing inappropriate drugs, adverse reactions, and suggested alternatives. Screening Tool to Alert doctors to the Right Treatment (START) has 22 criteria, also organized by body system, alerting physicians to appropriate treatment for older adults.

124. D: First-generation antihistamines, such as diphenhydramine and chlorpheniramine, should be avoided in older adults as they may result in confusion and/or falls because of sedation and anticholinergic effects. Alternate drugs include cetirizine, fexofenadine, loratadine, desloratadine, and levocetirizine. The other drugs are age- and dose-appropriate, although adverse effects (such as heart block and hypotension from metoprolol) may occur, so medications should be carefully monitored in older adults.

125. C: Young children between the ages of 1 and 4 are most at risk for unintentional injuries, so a class on preventing injuries is of most value. For example, the leading cause of death in young children is motor vehicle accidents—often as the result of the child being unrestrained, but some are pedestrian injuries. Toddlers are also at high risk of drowning and traumatic brain injuries.

Parents should be taught to keep pills, poisons, and caustic materials safeguarded out of reach of small children.

126. B: Dark-skinned individuals may exhibit cyanosis and pallor differently than Caucasians because changes in skin color and tone may be less noticeable. Cyanosis may be monitored by inspecting the client's conjunctiva, lips, palms, and soles of the feet. The palms and soles of the feet are often lighter in color than the rest of the client's skin. Pallor in an individual with brown skin may make the skin appear yellow-brown while pallor in an individual with very dark/black skin may make the skin appear ashen grey.

127. A: In an autosomal dominantly inherited disease, only a person who has inherited the defective gene and has the disease can pass on the disease to the next generation. There is no carrier state. Each pregnancy has a 50% risk of the child receiving the defective gene, although this does not necessarily mean that 50% of the children will have the disease. None or all may have it. Since there is no treatment and onset of symptoms is usually between ages 35 and 45, some people choose not to be tested, although many are tested at childbearing age.

128. B: Homeless clients are at high risk for noncompliance, so the best approach is to arrange for directly observed treatment (DOT) at the Salvation Army, as the client is more likely to cooperate if his routine is respected and few demands are placed on him. DOT allows the nurse administering the medication to assess the client for adverse effects and to observe the client actually taking the medication. Forcing the client into supervised housing may result in his running away, and providing a full course of treatment does not ensure the client takes the medication or allow for evaluation of adverse effects.

129. D: While all psychological/psychiatric disorders may put an older adult at increased risk after discharge from an inpatient facility, older adults are especially susceptible to depression, so a current diagnosis of depression or a history of depression places the client at increased risk. Clients should be screened for depression and appropriate treatment and support provided. The client must be assessed for the need for psychiatric care, and after-discharge caregivers should be aware of the client's needs. A support system should be identified.

130. C: The "iron triangle" comprises (1) the executive agency responsible for a policy area, (2) Congress and Congressional committees and subcommittees, and (3) interest groups/lobbyists. Organized interest groups, such as the American Nurses Association and the American Hospital Association have an advantage over individuals because they have resources and influence and are able to promote policy goals for their members and for the profession. They may provide education and conduct media campaigns to draw attention to issues.

131. B: According to Kingdon's Model of Policy Formulation, a possible solution is required before a problem is placed on the agenda in the problem stream. The model includes three streams:

- Problem: Crisis, feedback, various indicators that a problem exists.
- Policy: Matching the best of alternate solutions to the problem, considering technical feasibility and financial feasibility.
- Political Circumstances: Legislative realities/support, public knowledge, lobbying, media reports, political will to carry through with development of new policy.

132. A: One of the most serious current issues facing the nursing profession is a shortage of nurses. The average age of nurses is now 46 with about half nearing retirement age. Even if more students are interested in entering nursing programs, admission is often restricted. While lower nurse-patient ratios are reflected in better client outcomes, the nursing shortage is forcing some organizations to utilize more unlicensed assistive personnel and forcing nurses to work long hours.

133. D: When a sentinel event occurs, such as a behavioral health client who has received 24 hours per day care and commits suicide within 72 hours of discharge, then the facility must carry out a root-cause analysis to try to determine where in the processes an error might have occurred that resulted in the sentinel event. Once cause is determined, the facility is expected to develop an action plan to prevent further such events. The Joint Commission encourages organizations to report sentinel events but does not require they do so.

134. C: Lateral integration may refer to integration of services to clients between different settings and/or between different disciplines. In both cases, the role of the CNL is central to ensuring that client's needs are assessed and met and that these needs are communicated to all parties involved in client care. A primary goal is to ensure continuity of care and client safely without lapses in service. The CNL serves as an advocate for the client throughout the continuum of care.

135. A: The CNL should ask the ethics committee for guidance. While parents have a legal right to continue treatment, forcing a child to have treatment that will be ultimately futile presents an ethical dilemma. This is an appropriate issue for the ethics committee because the client wants one thing and the parents another; the client, while still a minor, is old enough to understand the full implications of his choice. The ethics committee can meet with those involved to try to reach a resolution.

136. C: Kohlberg's process of moral development (1971) was proposed for children but can be applied to adults as well. It comprises 3 levels:

- Preconventional: Person determines whether something is good or bad depending on consequences and does not question authority but acts to avoid punishment and does not understand underlying moral codes.
- Conventional: Person wants approval of others and wants to conform to the values of those in his/her group, responding to peer pressure.
- Post-conventional: Person understands personal responsibilities and societal expectations.

137. B: The American Hospital Association's Patient Care Partnership replaces the Patient Care Bill of Rights (2008) and states that clients should expect respect for values and spiritual beliefs. Other expectations include high quality care but does not specify how that will be provided, a clean and safe environment, personal involvement in care and decision making, protection of personal privacy, assistance with billing and insurance claims although not fair pricing, and discharge planning, including sources of care for follow-up treatment.

138. B: As part of the role of mentor, CNL should ask the nurse to call the physician and report the observations. Clients are often quite stressed about surgery and may forget what the physician has discussed with them, so the CNL should explain that the team member shouldn't assume that the physician is at fault but should report the findings so that the physician can speak with the client and answer any questions that the client may have.

139. A: The primary responsibility of an ethics committee is to provide guidance. The members may represent a number of different disciplines (physicians, nurses, administrators, allied health professionals) as well as community members, such as ministers, and should be knowledgeable about ethics and ethical odes, healthcare regulations, and privacy issues. The ethics committee may provide consultation to staff members, clients, and family who have questions about ethical issues. They may also help to facilitate communication and resolution of issues.

140. D: During the alert phase of a pandemic, risk assessment is critical. The four phases of a pandemic include:

- Interpandemic: This is the timer period between pandemics, during which people should begin risk assessment and make preparations (such as stockpiling antiviral drugs).
- Alert: A new strain or subtype has been identified, so people must be on alert for signs that the disease is spreading, carrying out increased local, national, and international risk assessment.
- Pandemic: The disease spreads internationally but the speed and spread may vary widely depending on multiple factors.
- Transition: The global risk decreases and activities are reduced.

141. C: The functional organization form divides departments by discipline (nurses, physical therapists, laboratory personnel) with each department developing its own hierarchical structure, polices, and procedures. With the parallel form, some services are shared across functional departments, such as human resources and rapid response teams. With program form, disciplines are integrated and departments formed with a special focus, such as women's health or rehabilitation. With matrix form, both functional and program forms overlap, so, for example, staff members report to both supervisors.

142. B: Ideally, the CNL would include the staff in decision-making, but if the CNL has made a decision based on valid research, the CNL should announce the decision, providing evidence-based rationale and establishing evaluation procedures so that staff members have some mechanism for feedback. If the CNL asks for input but ignores it, staff members may feel manipulated and may lose trust in the CNL. While voting sounds like a good plan, the CNL is responsible for improving client outcomes, and staff members may be more concerned with maintaining the status quo.

143. D: Return on investment (ROI) is a method used to estimate the value and cost of an investment, such as the purchase of new equipment. To calculate the productivity advantage in dollars, the CNL must multiply the yearly cost for the employee times the percentage of time (in decimals) that the employee will use the equipment times the percentage (in decimals) of estimated increased efficiency:

100,000 X 0.25 X 0.25 = $6,250.

144. D: When calculating the ROI, the CNL must first calculate the productivity advantage in dollars, in this case $6,250. Then, to calculate the number of months required to pay for the equipment, the CNL must divide the cost of equipment/training by the productivity advantage and multiply it by 12 (the number of months in a year):

50,000/6,250 = 8 x 12 = 96 months.

Because most equipment is outdated within 3 to 5 years, the purchase of this equipment may not be cost-effective if ROI is a primary concern.

145. A: In a disease management program, the initial step is to determine the population identification processes as well as selection criteria, taking into consideration risk assessment and risk stratification. Care should be provided through the use of evidence-based practice guidelines in a collaborative practice model. Client education for self-management should include primary prevention, behavior modification, and measures of compliance. Outcomes measurement, evaluation, and management must be planned for as well as routine reporting and feedback to all parties, including the client.

146. C: The four dimensions of nursing intensity include (1) illness severity, (2) dependency on nursing care, (3) complexity of condition, and (4) time necessary to provide care. The Patient Intensity for Nursing Index (PINI) is a classification system that considers both patient acuity and the need for nursing intervention. Each dimension has 10 different items that are scored on a scale of one to four with time loading calculated based on the scores of the first three dimensions.

147. A: When analyzing the effects of an intervention on outcomes in a varied population of clients, risk adjustment is a critical element because failure to consider relevant differences in clients can invalidate the outcomes. For example, if the client population includes those with and without co-morbidities as well as young clients and geriatric clients, then health issues or age may be more of a factor in outcomes than the intervention that is to be measured. Risk adjustment can be quite complicated.

148. D: A transformational leader makes team members feel important and value their work. The transformational leader models expected behavior and encourages and motivates staff. According to Bass (1998), the four primary components of a transformational leader are:

- Individualized consideration: The leader serves as a mentor and attends to the needs of the individuals.
- Charisma/Idealized influence: The leader models behavior that others try to emulate.
- Intellectual stimulation: The leader encourages creative solutions and supports staff, avoiding public criticism.
- Inspirational motivation: The leader promotes an inspiring vision that motivates staff members to take action.

149. A: Assigning clients according to numbers rarely results in an equitable case load, so changing to a client-acuity staffing pattern is probably the most effective change. Various methods can be used to classify clients, taking into consideration the number of care hours a client is likely to need and assigning clients to nurses accordingly, so nurses may have varying numbers of clients for whom they are responsible. Acuity-based staffing is sometimes used across an organization, so that staffing may fluctuate on a unit depending on the acuity of the clients.

150. A: Conflict resolution strategies include:

- Avoiding: Refusing to acknowledge conflict and wanting to leave well enough alone.
- Smoothing over/Reassuring: Surface harmony is maintained by using verbal communication to calm those in conflict.
- Withholding/Withdrawing: One party to the conflict withdraws, leaving the conflict unresolved but decreasing tension.
- Accommodating: The one with lesser power accedes to the one with greater power.

How to Overcome Test Anxiety

Just the thought of taking a test is enough to make most people a little nervous. A test is an important event that can have a long-term impact on your future, so it's important to take it seriously and it's natural to feel anxious about performing well. But just because anxiety is normal, that doesn't mean that it's helpful in test taking, or that you should simply accept it as part of your life. Anxiety can have a variety of effects. These effects can be mild, like making you feel slightly nervous, or severe, like blocking your ability to focus or remember even a simple detail.

If you experience test anxiety—whether severe or mild—it's important to know how to beat it. To discover this, first you need to understand what causes test anxiety.

Causes of Test Anxiety

While we often think of anxiety as an uncontrollable emotional state, it can actually be caused by simple, practical things. One of the most common causes of test anxiety is that a person does not feel adequately prepared for their test. This feeling can be the result of many different issues such as poor study habits or lack of organization, but the most common culprit is time management. Starting to study too late, failing to organize your study time to cover all of the material, or being distracted while you study will mean that you're not well prepared for the test. This may lead to cramming the night before, which will cause you to be physically and mentally exhausted for the test. Poor time management also contributes to feelings of stress, fear, and hopelessness as you realize you are not well prepared but don't know what to do about it.

Other times, test anxiety is not related to your preparation for the test but comes from unresolved fear. This may be a past failure on a test, or poor performance on tests in general. It may come from comparing yourself to others who seem to be performing better or from the stress of living up to expectations. Anxiety may be driven by fears of the future—how failure on this test would affect your educational and career goals. These fears are often completely irrational, but they can still negatively impact your test performance.

Elements of Test Anxiety

As mentioned earlier, test anxiety is considered to be an emotional state, but it has physical and mental components as well. Sometimes you may not even realize that you are suffering from test anxiety until you notice the physical symptoms. These can include trembling hands, rapid heartbeat, sweating, nausea, and tense muscles. Extreme anxiety may lead to fainting or vomiting. Obviously, any of these symptoms can have a negative impact on testing. It is important to recognize them as soon as they begin to occur so that you can address the problem before it damages your performance.

The mental components of test anxiety include trouble focusing and inability to remember learned information. During a test, your mind is on high alert, which can help you recall information and stay focused for an extended period of time. However, anxiety interferes with your mind's natural processes, causing you to blank out, even on the questions you know well. The strain of testing during anxiety makes it difficult to stay focused, especially on a test that may take several hours. Extreme anxiety can take a huge mental toll, making it difficult not only to recall test information but even to understand the test questions or pull your thoughts together.

Effects of Test Anxiety

Test anxiety is like a disease—if left untreated, it will get progressively worse. Anxiety leads to poor performance, and this reinforces the feelings of fear and failure, which in turn lead to poor performances on subsequent tests. It can grow from a mild nervousness to a crippling condition. If allowed to progress, test anxiety can have a big impact on your schooling, and consequently on your future.

Test anxiety can spread to other parts of your life. Anxiety on tests can become anxiety in any stressful situation, and blanking on a test can turn into panicking in a job situation. But fortunately, you don't have to let anxiety rule your testing and determine your grades. There are a number of relatively simple steps you can take to move past anxiety and function normally on a test and in the rest of life.

Physical Steps for Beating Test Anxiety

While test anxiety is a serious problem, the good news is that it can be overcome. It doesn't have to control your ability to think and remember information. While it may take time, you can begin taking steps today to beat anxiety.

Just as your first hint that you may be struggling with anxiety comes from the physical symptoms, the first step to treating it is also physical. Rest is crucial for having a clear, strong mind. If you are tired, it is much easier to give in to anxiety. But if you establish good sleep habits, your body and mind will be ready to perform optimally, without the strain of exhaustion. Additionally, sleeping well helps you to retain information better, so you're more likely to recall the answers when you see the test questions.

Getting good sleep means more than going to bed on time. It's important to allow your brain time to relax. Take study breaks from time to time so it doesn't get overworked, and don't study right before bed. Take time to rest your mind before trying to rest your body, or you may find it difficult to fall asleep.

Along with sleep, other aspects of physical health are important in preparing for a test. Good nutrition is vital for good brain function. Sugary foods and drinks may give a burst of energy but this burst is followed by a crash, both physically and emotionally. Instead, fuel your body with protein and vitamin-rich foods.

Also, drink plenty of water. Dehydration can lead to headaches and exhaustion, especially if your brain is already under stress from the rigors of the test. Particularly if your test is a long one, drink water during the breaks. And if possible, take an energy-boosting snack to eat between sections.

Along with sleep and diet, a third important part of physical health is exercise. Maintaining a steady workout schedule is helpful, but even taking 5-minute study breaks to walk can help get your blood pumping faster and clear your head. Exercise also releases endorphins, which contribute to a positive feeling and can help combat test anxiety.

When you nurture your physical health, you are also contributing to your mental health. If your body is healthy, your mind is much more likely to be healthy as well. So take time to rest, nourish your body with healthy food and water, and get moving as much as possible. Taking these physical steps will make you stronger and more able to take the mental steps necessary to overcome test anxiety.

Mental Steps for Beating Test Anxiety

Working on the mental side of test anxiety can be more challenging, but as with the physical side, there are clear steps you can take to overcome it. As mentioned earlier, test anxiety often stems from lack of preparation, so the obvious solution is to prepare for the test. Effective studying may be the most important weapon you have for beating test anxiety, but you can and should employ several other mental tools to combat fear.

First, boost your confidence by reminding yourself of past success—tests or projects that you aced. If you're putting as much effort into preparing for this test as you did for those, there's no reason you should expect to fail here. Work hard to prepare; then trust your preparation.

Second, surround yourself with encouraging people. It can be helpful to find a study group, but be sure that the people you're around will encourage a positive attitude. If you spend time with others who are anxious or cynical, this will only contribute to your own anxiety. Look for others who are motivated to study hard from a desire to succeed, not from a fear of failure.

Third, reward yourself. A test is physically and mentally tiring, even without anxiety, and it can be helpful to have something to look forward to. Plan an activity following the test, regardless of the outcome, such as going to a movie or getting ice cream.

When you are taking the test, if you find yourself beginning to feel anxious, remind yourself that you know the material. Visualize successfully completing the test. Then take a few deep, relaxing breaths and return to it. Work through the questions carefully but with confidence, knowing that you are capable of succeeding.

Developing a healthy mental approach to test taking will also aid in other areas of life. Test anxiety affects more than just the actual test—it can be damaging to your mental health and even contribute to depression. It's important to beat test anxiety before it becomes a problem for more than testing.

Study Strategy

Being prepared for the test is necessary to combat anxiety, but what does being prepared look like? You may study for hours on end and still not feel prepared. What you need is a strategy for test prep. The next few pages outline our recommended steps to help you plan out and conquer the challenge of preparation.

STEP 1: SCOPE OUT THE TEST

Learn everything you can about the format (multiple choice, essay, etc.) and what will be on the test. Gather any study materials, course outlines, or sample exams that may be available. Not only will this help you to prepare, but knowing what to expect can help to alleviate test anxiety.

STEP 2: MAP OUT THE MATERIAL

Look through the textbook or study guide and make note of how many chapters or sections it has. Then divide these over the time you have. For example, if a book has 15 chapters and you have five days to study, you need to cover three chapters each day. Even better, if you have the time, leave an extra day at the end for overall review after you have gone through the material in depth.

If time is limited, you may need to prioritize the material. Look through it and make note of which sections you think you already have a good grasp on, and which need review. While you are studying, skim quickly through the familiar sections and take more time on the challenging parts.

Write out your plan so you don't get lost as you go. Having a written plan also helps you feel more in control of the study, so anxiety is less likely to arise from feeling overwhelmed at the amount to cover.

STEP 3: GATHER YOUR TOOLS

Decide what study method works best for you. Do you prefer to highlight in the book as you study and then go back over the highlighted portions? Or do you type out notes of the important information? Or is it helpful to make flashcards that you can carry with you? Assemble the pens, index cards, highlighters, post-it notes, and any other materials you may need so you won't be distracted by getting up to find things while you study.

If you're having a hard time retaining the information or organizing your notes, experiment with different methods. For example, try color-coding by subject with colored pens, highlighters, or post-it notes. If you learn better by hearing, try recording yourself reading your notes so you can listen while in the car, working out, or simply sitting at your desk. Ask a friend to quiz you from your flashcards, or try teaching someone the material to solidify it in your mind.

STEP 4: CREATE YOUR ENVIRONMENT

It's important to avoid distractions while you study. This includes both the obvious distractions like visitors and the subtle distractions like an uncomfortable chair (or a too-comfortable couch that makes you want to fall asleep). Set up the best study environment possible: good lighting and a comfortable work area. If background music helps you focus, you may want to turn it on, but otherwise keep the room quiet. If you are using a computer to take notes, be sure you don't have any other windows open, especially applications like social media, games, or anything else that could distract you. Silence your phone and turn off notifications. Be sure to keep water close by so you stay hydrated while you study (but avoid unhealthy drinks and snacks).

Also, take into account the best time of day to study. Are you freshest first thing in the morning? Try to set aside some time then to work through the material. Is your mind clearer in the afternoon or evening? Schedule your study session then. Another method is to study at the same time of day that you will take the test, so that your brain gets used to working on the material at that time and will be ready to focus at test time.

STEP 5: STUDY!

Once you have done all the study preparation, it's time to settle into the actual studying. Sit down, take a few moments to settle your mind so you can focus, and begin to follow your study plan. Don't give in to distractions or let yourself procrastinate. This is your time to prepare so you'll be ready to fearlessly approach the test. Make the most of the time and stay focused.

Of course, you don't want to burn out. If you study too long you may find that you're not retaining the information very well. Take regular study breaks. For example, taking five minutes out of every hour to walk briskly, breathing deeply and swinging your arms, can help your mind stay fresh.

As you get to the end of each chapter or section, it's a good idea to do a quick review. Remind yourself of what you learned and work on any difficult parts. When you feel that you've mastered the material, move on to the next part. At the end of your study session, briefly skim through your notes again.

But while review is helpful, cramming last minute is NOT. If at all possible, work ahead so that you won't need to fit all your study into the last day. Cramming overloads your brain with more information than it can process and retain, and your tired mind may struggle to recall even previously learned information when it is overwhelmed with last-minute study. Also, the urgent nature of cramming and the stress placed on your brain contribute to anxiety. You'll be more likely to go to the test feeling unprepared and having trouble thinking clearly.

So don't cram, and don't stay up late before the test, even just to review your notes at a leisurely pace. Your brain needs rest more than it needs to go over the information again. In fact, plan to finish your studies by noon or early afternoon the day before the test. Give your brain the rest of the day to relax or focus on other things, and get a good night's sleep. Then you will be fresh for the test and better able to recall what you've studied.

STEP 6: TAKE A PRACTICE TEST

Many courses offer sample tests, either online or in the study materials. This is an excellent resource to check whether you have mastered the material, as well as to prepare for the test format and environment.

Check the test format ahead of time: the number of questions, the type (multiple choice, free response, etc.), and the time limit. Then create a plan for working through them. For example, if you have 30 minutes to take a 60-question test, your limit is 30 seconds per question. Spend less time on the questions you know well so that you can take more time on the difficult ones.

If you have time to take several practice tests, take the first one open book, with no time limit. Work through the questions at your own pace and make sure you fully understand them. Gradually work up to taking a test under test conditions: sit at a desk with all study materials put away and set a timer. Pace yourself to make sure you finish the test with time to spare and go back to check your answers if you have time.

After each test, check your answers. On the questions you missed, be sure you understand why you missed them. Did you misread the question (tests can use tricky wording)? Did you forget the information? Or was it something you hadn't learned? Go back and study any shaky areas that the practice tests reveal.

Taking these tests not only helps with your grade, but also aids in combating test anxiety. If you're already used to the test conditions, you're less likely to worry about it, and working through tests until you're scoring well gives you a confidence boost. Go through the practice tests until you feel comfortable, and then you can go into the test knowing that you're ready for it.

Test Tips

On test day, you should be confident, knowing that you've prepared well and are ready to answer the questions. But aside from preparation, there are several test day strategies you can employ to maximize your performance.

First, as stated before, get a good night's sleep the night before the test (and for several nights before that, if possible). Go into the test with a fresh, alert mind rather than staying up late to study.

Try not to change too much about your normal routine on the day of the test. It's important to eat a nutritious breakfast, but if you normally don't eat breakfast at all, consider eating just a protein bar. If you're a coffee drinker, go ahead and have your normal coffee. Just make sure you time it so that the caffeine doesn't wear off right in the middle of your test. Avoid sugary beverages, and drink enough water to stay hydrated but not so much that you need a restroom break 10 minutes into the test. If your test isn't first thing in the morning, consider going for a walk or doing a light workout before the test to get your blood flowing.

Allow yourself enough time to get ready, and leave for the test with plenty of time to spare so you won't have the anxiety of scrambling to arrive in time. Another reason to be early is to select a good seat. It's helpful to sit away from doors and windows, which can be distracting. Find a good seat, get out your supplies, and settle your mind before the test begins.

When the test begins, start by going over the instructions carefully, even if you already know what to expect. Make sure you avoid any careless mistakes by following the directions.

Then begin working through the questions, pacing yourself as you've practiced. If you're not sure on an answer, don't spend too much time on it, and don't let it shake your confidence. Either skip it and come back later, or eliminate as many wrong answers as possible and guess among the remaining ones. Don't dwell on these questions as you continue—put them out of your mind and focus on what lies ahead.

Be sure to read all of the answer choices, even if you're sure the first one is the right answer. Sometimes you'll find a better one if you keep reading. But don't second-guess yourself if you do immediately know the answer. Your gut instinct is usually right. Don't let test anxiety rob you of the information you know.

If you have time at the end of the test (and if the test format allows), go back and review your answers. Be cautious about changing any, since your first instinct tends to be correct, but make sure you didn't misread any of the questions or accidentally mark the wrong answer choice. Look over any you skipped and make an educated guess.

At the end, leave the test feeling confident. You've done your best, so don't waste time worrying about your performance or wishing you could change anything. Instead, celebrate the successful completion of this test. And finally, use this test to learn how to deal with anxiety even better next time.

> **Review Video: Test Anxiety**
> Visit mometrix.com/academy and enter code: 100340

Important Qualification

Not all anxiety is created equal. If your test anxiety is causing major issues in your life beyond the classroom or testing center, or if you are experiencing troubling physical symptoms related to your anxiety, it may be a sign of a serious physiological or psychological condition. If this sounds like your situation, we strongly encourage you to seek professional help.

Additional Bonus Material

Due to our efforts to try to keep this book to a manageable length, we've created a link that will give you access to all of your additional bonus material:

mometrix.com/bonus948/clinnurselead